Perfect Health FOR **Kids**

Perfect Health

FOR Kids

Ten Ayurvedic Health Secrets
Every Parent Must Know

DR. JOHN DOUILLARD

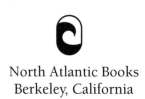

North Atlantic Books
Berkeley, California

Published by
North Atlantic Books
P.O. Box 12327
Berkeley, California 94712

Cover and Book design by Suzanne Albertson
Printed in Canada

Perfect Health for Kids: Ten Ayurvedic Health Secrets Every Parent Should Know is sponsored by the Society for the Study of Native Arts and Sciences, a nonprofit educational corporation whose goals are to develop an educational and crosscultural perspective linking various scientific, social, and artistic fields; to nurture a holistic view of arts, sciences, humanities, and healing; and to publish and distribute literature on the relationship of mind, body, and nature.

North Atlantic Books' publications are available through most bookstores. For further information, call 800-337-2665 or visit our website at www.northatlanticbooks.com.

Substantial discounts on bulk quantities are available to corporations, professional associations, and other organizations. For details and discount information, contact our special sales department.

Library of Congress Cataloging-in-Publication Data

Douillard, John.
    Perfect health for kids : ten ayurvedic health secrets every parent
    should know / by John Douillard.
        p. cm.
    ISBN 1-55643-477-4
    1. Children—Health and hygiene. 2. Medicine, Ayurvedic. I. Title:
    Ten ayurvedic healing secrets every parent should know. II. Title.
    RJ61.D724 2003
    613'.0432—dc22
                                            2003017003

    1   2   3   4   5   6   7   8   9   TRANS   09   08   07   06   05   04

Acknowledgments

I am truly blessed in this life to have such a wonderful family of six children and a loving and beautiful wife. Without them, I could not have written this book.

I want to thank Felicia Tomasko for her help with editing the Ayurveda and science aspects of the book, and Kate Fotopoulos for copyediting and catching all the little details that might have slipped through the cracks. Thanks to Samara Frame for her administrative support.

Thank you to Brooke Warner, Richard Grossinger, and everyone at my new publisher, North Atlantic Books.

Thank you to all my patients and students who continually show me and my family the way to Perfect Health.

Table of Contents

Introduction

In America, before the general use of antibiotics in the 1940s, parents raised their children proactively. They did not wait until their children were sick; kids were treated each day while they were healthy as a part of their normal daily routine. Nature provided the medicines. Even today, 80% of our pharmaceutical drugs come directly from, are derived from, or are copied from natural substances. The seasonal harvest of foods and herbs was always the medicine of the day. Throughout history, people were connected to their neighborhood farmer via the local harvest and were therefore attuned to and lived in harmony with the rhythms and cycles of the land. In this book, *Perfect Health for Kids,* I will reintroduce the now lost wisdom that once kept our kids healthy.

During my post-graduate studies in Ayurvedic medicine, I realized that what I was learning as a part of this 5,000-year-old system of medicine was fundamentally the same as what we in America have lost in our own medical tradition. As we have focused on hunting down the cures for diseases, we have slowly forgotten the fabrics of good health that this "science of life" so clearly deemed paramount. Ayurveda, which means "science of life," emphasized prevention by proactively treating people when they were healthy and focusing on *who* had the disease rather than on the disease itself.

While raising my six children and practicing natural medicine with kids for 18 years, I have rediscovered ten ancient healing secrets that will change how you raise your children. You will effortlessly treat your kids while they are healthy, and identify and take care of a cold weeks before it arises. You will learn the early warning signs of an illness-in-the-making and how to "inspect" your kids each morning for those signs.

One of the cornerstones of Ayurveda explained in the book is that each child is unique. Each has constitutional differences that explain the child's unique health, behavior and emotional make-up.

1

I will discuss how, when, and what to feed your children, the amount of pure water (not soda pop) they should drink, the insidious toxic chemical levels in your home, and other factors that can directly affect your children's health and well-being. You will learn what activities and times of year make your children more susceptible to getting sick and what to do about it. I will introduce you to my "Lazy Susan" of natural medicines, which you can choose from each day to address each of your children's different needs. *Perfect Health for Kids* would be remiss if it didn't address the emotional health and human potential of your children. I will introduce effective tools you can use to access and support your children's emotional health, and will discuss the importance of "play" for both parents and children.

Ayurvedic medicine was originally used as preparation for achieving full human potential. Keeping a child in good physical, mental and emotional health is a prerequisite for a successful spiritual practice later in life. While *Perfect Health for Kids* is all about the day-to-day tools a parent will need to keep their child healthy, it is also building a foundation for children to develop into well-balanced physical, emotional and spiritual beings. This knowledge will change your life as a parent and protect the lives of your children—it did mine, and for that I am very grateful.

While many of the *Perfect Health for Kids* principles will work for adults, I highly recommend parents read the best-selling book *Perfect Health* by Dr. Deepak Chopra. This comprehensive mind-body guide to Ayurvedic medicine is written for adults and elucidates the road to optimal health.

Chapter 1

"Knowledge": A Parent's Best Medicine

In the past 70 years we have seen miraculous developments in our health care system. In this relatively short time span we have seen the practice of modern medicine make significant advances, from the development and widespread use of the magic bullets of life-saving penicillin and other antibiotics in the 1940s, to the present when many patients walk out of a hospital the day they have heart surgery. These are incredible times in the health care field and the next decades promise to bring even more innovations. Health care is still a work in progress and doctors still call the art and science of medicine "practice" for a reason. The practice of modern medicine is changing and evolving as the acceptance of complementary and alternative medicine becomes more widespread.

We have all rightfully become fascinated by the science and technology of modern health care. It is important, however, that this fascination not blind us from the information contained in the healing pearls of health care wisdom that were a part of mainstream American awareness just 50 years ago. This knowledge, while almost lost in today's society, is still practiced in many traditional cultures worldwide. I did my post-graduate work in Ayurvedic healing—one of the world's oldest systems of medicine still practiced on this planet today. Ayurveda is India's 5,000-year-old medical tradition. Ayurveda, the "science of life," is the study of life, not disease.

I started teaching Ayurveda in the United States in 1987 and have since spent most of my time translating this still intact science of life into our American culture, which until recently incorporated many of the same traditions and practices as Ayurveda. In this book I will introduce many simple, effective, and logical health care concepts that are drawn from the science of Ayurveda. I am not introducing lifestyle changes that will turn anyone's life upside down; rather I aim to make life simpler for parents and simultaneously healthier for children (and the entire family).

I have been troubleshooting and fine-tuning the integration of these concepts into the modern American way of life with my six children with the belief that if I alienate my own kids from the mainstream culture, they will in time rebel against everything I am trying to teach them. As a result, my kids have what I believe to be a healthy balance between being a part of this mainstream American culture and maintaining good health. Consequently, my kids are generally healthy and they rarely get sick. They have embraced the tenets of good health and appreciate the balance my wife and I have offered them through this lifestyle. We have not chosen a lifestyle of extremes; we drink soda pop and eat pizza and Mac 'n' Cheese. But when we eat these types of foods, the kids realize it is a treat and not a daily event.

The 51% Rule

I do not expect parents to feel obliged to implement every one of these Ayurvedic health secrets immediately into their family lives for the advice in this book to be effective. Please incorporate what I call the "51% Rule." This means that if you integrate these concepts most of the time, such as four days out of seven, you will be living a healthier lifestyle the majority of your life—51% of your life at least. As you incorporate these changes, you and your children will feel healthier. Positive results will convince you to make the suggested adjustments to your lifestyle because it is your choice to do so, not because of some dogma from a book.

Helpful Hint! You may not choose to implement this information right away; it may be years before you feel ready to make these changes. Today we may just be planting seeds which might take years to germinate.

The Culture

Before I discuss the secrets to raising kids in perfect health, let's examine the culture we live in. On average, school-age children in America experience eight to ten colds a year, according to *The Children's Hospital Guide to Your Child's Health and Development*, and American pediatricians prescribe over $500 million of antibiotics a year to fight them. According to recent Congressional hearings, up to 60% of those antibiotics are misprescribed, and therefore ineffective. In spite of this, prescriptions for young children have risen by a staggering 51% over the past 15 years. The U.S. Centers for Disease Control and Prevention (CDC) strongly urge physicians to use antibiotics only when absolutely necessary. Campaigns to this effect have had some impact. A 2003 survey in the *Annals of Internal Medicine* reports that throughout the 1990s doctors cut back on the prescription of antibiotics.

This seems heartening, but the report also reveals that most of the antibiotics prescribed in the U.S. are stronger, broad-spectrum antibiotics that are more expensive, have more side effects, and should be reserved for bacteria that cause severe infections rather than the "garden-variety respiratory tract infections" treated in the doctor's office. As of 1999, 40% of the antibiotics prescribed to children were broad-spectrum, which are still misprescribed for colds and other viruses. In fact, 14% of children given broad-spectrum antibiotics were diagnosed with a common cold or viral infection. Prescriptions given out for the common cold were even higher. Antibiotics given to treat the common cold or a virus will be ineffective and are therefore unnecessary.

> One of the difficult things about the antibiotic controversy is that there are no current widely accepted alternative solutions.

Something is wrong with this situation, and parents know it. Kids are getting sicker, bacteria are getting stronger, and effective treatments are slowly vanishing.

In our family, with six children under the age of 15, chronic colds have been declared an "unacceptable behavior." By "colds" I mean severe, debilitating, lingering colds with fever, chills, and doctor bills. Although it seems hard to believe, mild colds which last only two to three days build strong immune systems, actually benefitting a child. The severity of a child's cold or illness largely lays in the hands of us parents, not doctors.

In our house, with six kids and two adults under the same roof, we just can't afford to do colds. For example, if one kid gets a cold, he or she might be out of school for a week or two. If it is contagious, as most colds are, somewhere during the second week of the kid's cold, another kid comes down with the same cold, and there goes another two weeks. If this cold makes its way through every kid and adult in the house, and each cold lasts, let's say, one week per person, then it's eight weeks before the Douillard family is finally healthy again. Between doctor visits, baby sitters, and kids staying home sick, we would have no life for two months. If each of our kids caught only six colds a year, which represents the low end of the national average, our family would experience continual runny noses, fevers, and doctor visits for the entire year. Even if each cold lasted only a couple of days, we are talking about an unacceptable number of sick days. In our case, it was an absolute necessity to learn how to raise six healthy children.

Lucas and the Never-Ending Cold

My own kids are not the only ones I need to keep healthy. Patients of mine bring their children and tell me an all-too-familiar story. A recent example of this story came from an 8-year-old boy named Lucas who came to see me complaining of a chronic cold.

Four months prior to visiting my office, Lucas came down with an earache, a fever, and a cold. His parents had taken him to a doctor who prescribed antibiotics that seemed to work; within a week or so he was healthy and back to school. Then about two or three weeks later, his earache was back, his nose started running, and he began to cough. Again he was off to the doctor's office where they prescribed a more powerful course of antibiotics. The same cycle repeated itself: first he would get better and then he became worse. It became very clear that the antibiotics were getting Lucas out of immediate danger from the acute infection, but they were not helping him stay well. After one more course of antibiotics, now four months since the first cold, Lucas's mom heard me on my radio show talking about how to prevent colds in kids, so she brought him in.

"The best medicine for an earache, cold, or flu," I told Lucas's mom, "is to prevent it from happening. Let's learn how to treat Lucas when he is healthy and keep him that way." This may sound ridiculous because in our society we are taught to focus on treating the infection once it has already occurred, while little is ever mentioned about how to prevent it. Antibiotics will likely kill Lucas's infection, but a crucial question always remains: what is causing this infection to reoccur, and how can we treat the underlying cause? By understanding the underlying cause of colds, earaches, asthma, and allergies, there is a lot we can do to prevent the common cold and its companions.

Parents Must Get Involved

In my practice, I have noticed that many parents are starting to resist taking their kids to a medical doctor when they catch a cold because they worry that it will result in more antibiotics and nothing else, just like Lucas's situation. It is now becoming common knowledge that the overuse of antibiotics breeds resistant strains of bacteria and that antibiotics themselves are not always the best solution for kids due to their known side effects. Therefore, it is unsurprising that many parents are resisting the use of antibiotics to treat their child's illnesses. However, it's important to remember that antibiotics can save lives when a child becomes severely ill and is in life-threatening danger from a bacterial infection. The bottom line is that antibiotics are appropriate for certain illnesses, but should not be overprescribed.

If you have a small child who's sick and you are debating whether or not to take him or her to the doctor's office, just do it. It's dangerous to resist taking your child to a doctor because you think antibiotics are bad. I know too many patients who now, after the fact, wish they hadn't had this mindset. If you don't want your child to take antibiotics, make sure you are making an informed decision. There is no better person to help you make that decision than your doctor or primary health care practitioner. Remember that doctors are not always right, though. Parents should go to the doctor armed with the right questions so that when their child is prescribed a medication, it can be accepted or rejected based on a decision made by both the parent and the doctor.

Don't be bashful when asking your doctor questions about natural medicine alternatives. You are not alone: 42% of Americans are using complementary and alternative medicine (CAM) practitioners and spending $30 billion a year on natural health care. Most doctors will not be offended if you ask questions about alternatives; in fact, 52% of medical doctors now use complementary and alternative medicine for their own personal care.

Here are some of the more general questions you should think to ask when taking your child to a doctor:

Is the cold bacterial or viral?
 ○ Antibiotics will treat only bacterial infections.

If my child doesn't take the medication, what is worst that can happen?
 ○ Make sure the medication is absolutely necessary. Sometimes doctors feel they should prescribe something even when studies show the condition will heal on its own just as quickly.

Are there any natural substances that will help?

○ More and more doctors prescribe natural medicines for milder conditions. Patients are an educational resource and motivating factor for doctors. They will have more incentive to broaden their knowledge base if you come with questions.

What are the side effects of the medication?

○ Every medication has a list of side effects that is enclosed as a package insert. The prescribing doctor should know if the medication is contraindicated for your child for any reason and should ensure that there are no harmful side effects.

Will taking this medication *now* make my child more susceptible to either the same or another illness in the future?

○ Doctors are aware that medications can have miraculous results for symptom eradication but can also make the child more susceptible to the same or other illnesses in the future, which is why more doctors are turning to natural medicines.

If we run all these tests and spend all this money, will the results change what you would prescribe?

○ It is important to know before you spend the money on a series of tests whether the test results will alter decisions about the treatment. If you know that the possible treatment is unacceptable for you—or the doctor will prescribe the treatment regardless—then you might want to reconsider your options.

When looking for a doctor for your child's condition there are four critical questions to ask:

1. Does the practitioner treat my child's specific condition?
2. How frequently does the practitioner treat my child's specific condition?
3. What training and specialized equipment does the practitioner have to treat my child's specific condition?
4. How successful has the practitioner been in treating my child's specific condition?

There are also patient-doctor referral services that can help. A new company called *4 Healing* provides a service that will match your child's condition with a medical doctor or CAM practicitioner in your area who has treated that condition successfully on a regular basis. See their website at www.4Healing.com.

Be an Educated User

Too many medical doctors over-prescribe antibiotics without getting a confirmed diagnosis of a bacterial infection. This overuse, coupled with the fact that many patients fail to finish their prescriptions, has led to a significant increase in the number of antibiotic-resistant strains of bacteria. This over-prescription also has serious consequences for individuals and the environment.

Any bacteria that is exposed to antibiotics and survives the assault then passes their resistance onto their offspring. Because bacteria multiply rapidly and have short generation times, they pass that resistance onto thousands of other bacteria in incredibly short periods of time. In one study, a single bacterium produced more than a million offspring in ten hours. If this bacterium survived an antibiotic attack, it could pass on the advantage to millions of offspring in a matter of hours. Continued overuse and misuse of antibiotics will only exacerbate this situation.

Why Do Some People Get Infected While Others Do Not?

This question is a that has been debated heatedly over time. Louis Pasteur and Claude Bernard famously argued over this question in the nineteenth century. Pasteur is the father and champion of the germ theory of modern medicine He identified anthrax, encouraged doctors to wash their hands between patients, and recommended the heating of milk (pasteurization) to kill bacteria. Bernard is considered to be the father of modern physiology. He believed that it is something about the individual that determines whether or not they will become infected with a pathogen. He said, "Illnesses hover constantly above us, their seeds blown by the wind, but they do not set in the terrain unless the terrain is ready to receive them."

Bernard and Pasteur fought over this issue throughout their lives, until Pasteur's famous deathbed confession when he said that it is the "soil, not the seed," which is most responsible for disease. And he conceded the fight to Bernard, saying, "I have been wrong. The germ is nothing. The terrain is everything."

The terrain is that of our own bodies, and the seeds are the pathogenic microorganisms that inhabit our environment. But to say that the germ is nothing is not quite right. We have seen the power of microorganisms to infect us and to spread from person to person. We have witnessed new diseases emerge in our time. The 2003 spread of Sudden Acute Respiratory Syndrome (SARS) was an example of a disease that passes from person to person. But even with this syndrome, not everyone who was exposed to the virus contracted the disease. There was still the interaction of the seeds and the soil.

What I have found in my clinical research with my family and patients, and one of the key points of this book, is that there are a wealth of things we can all do to keep ourselves healthy and therefore less susceptible to infection.

The first thing we can do is to have the basic understanding that any treatment, whether it is preventive or therapeutic, must be targeted at the needs of the individual not the symptoms. The concerned parent and doctor should not ask, "What is the treatment for the *disease*?" but rather, "How do we treat the individual who has the disease?" The longer we focus on suppressing symptoms, the more tenacious the cause of the disease becomes, and the more difficult it can become to treat effectively.

Second, if we choose to go down the road of prophylactically using antibiotics to combat diseases like anthrax, we will likely hasten the development of much more potent and resistant strains of already lethal bacteria. An April 3, 2003, report by the CDC in the *New England Journal of Medicine* stated the alarming fact that one-third of all Americans host *Staphylococcus aureus* on their skin or in their nasal passages. Staph is the most common cause of skin infections and is resistant to all current antibiotics, including vancomycin, the strongest broad-spectrum antibiotic available. Antibiotics are ineffective against viral infections so it is important to ask your doctor if the infection is bacterial or viral. *The Journal of the American Medical Association* recently published a report stating that 90% of common upper-respiratory infections routinely treated with antibiotics are in fact viral rather than bacterial. Some doctors don't appreciate their patients asking a lot of questions, so it is your responsibility to find a doctor who you feel comfortable talking with. Good communication can save your child's life, as it did with one of mine—a story I tell in Chapter 9. Find a doctor who is up to date with the growing field of natural medicine and is aware of the pros and cons of antibiotics and commonly prescribed pharmaceutical drugs. Medical doctors are becoming more educated in the field of natural medicine, so keep checking in your area. I have trained over 2,000 medical doctors in Ayurveda, and the interest continues to rise. I am also on the faculty of The American Board of Holistic Medicine (ABHM), which is a good place to find a medical doctor certified in holistic health care. They can be found at www.amerboardholisticmed.org.

Parents Have Homework

When I first got the idea to write this book, we had raised four kids without using antibiotics, and at the time, our fifth child, an 8-month-old boy, was antibiotic-free. Not a bad track record, I thought: raising five kids without using antibiotics. I learned how to help kids like Lucas restore their health because of my front-line experience with my own six children and my young patients. Part of the key to this success is to never say never…even to antibiotics. As I have said before, each type of therapeutic treatment has its place. A closed mind is a dangerous mind.

> The real key to healthy children and the main focus of this book is to do our best to keep them from getting sick in the first place. If we could master that, the question of whether or not they should take antibiotics wouldn't even come up.

Will your child never catch a cold after you read this book? Absolutely not. In fact, as I mentioned earlier in this chapter, some mild colds are good for kids; they help develop strong broad-based immunity in the body. Eight to ten colds a year, on the other hand, are debilitating and dangerous. If you follow the prevention tips, though, when your child does get a cold it will not be nearly as severe nor last nearly as long. By following these suggestions, your child will catch only the mildest form of the cold: one that may last one or two days rather than one to two weeks. Antibiotics and doctor's visits will be dramatically reduced as you watch your child fight his or her own battles and build the strong immune system that is so crucial in these uncertain times.

I am not an extremist—my kids do not live in a glass bubble without pizza, candy, or Coke, although these foods are not the mainstay of their diet. I think you will find the simple measures in this book to be both logical and backed by common sense. If I tell you to avoid a food in a certain season, or not to eat it at a certain time of day, I will make sure you understand why. When you're finished reading, I hope will understand the reasons why kids get sick and why the simple Do's and Don'ts in this book make sense. Keeping kids healthy is not rocket science. As you will see, it is basic common sense put into practice.

We have twenty-four kids on our small cul-de-sac, and we watch as many of them continually go on and off antibiotics, year after year. We have five kids who play tackle on the lawn with the neighbors and who are in and out of classrooms, too. If being exposed to germs were the only cause of the common cold, we would be one sick family. As it turns out, though our kids are constantly exposed to germs, they typically do not get sick. Although you cannot keep your kids from being exposed to the so-called cold-causing germs, you can keep them healthy and strong enough to not succumb to the germs and subsequent illnesses.

I will list the ten Ayurvedic secrets that will keep your kids healthy, and they all require a little parental "super–vision." Once you learn the rules, and how to assess your kids on a daily and seasonal basis, keeping your kids healthy will be a snap. The side benefit of this knowledge is that it works for adults as well. The result is a healthier family.

As the autumn season progresses, just as the leaves get dry and brittle, we notice our skin becomes parched, stretched, and cracked; we feel our sinuses get dry and uncomfortable. If we allow our sinuses to become excessively dry, the mucous membranes in the nose become irritated. As a result, the sinuses begin to make more mucus to combat and soothe the dryness and irritation. This excessive production of mucus compromises the immune system's ability to fight against airborne bacteria or viruses. It also provides a breeding ground for pathogenic, disease-causing bacteria to proliferate. By this time we are into November and December, appropriately named Cold and Flu Season.

If we notice nature and its harvest in the fall and winter, we see that squirrels gather lots of nuts. It is clear that the nuts, grains, root vegetables, and meats, which are more available in the winter, provide the fat and protein needed to help insulate and lubricate the mucous membranes of the sinuses, preventing them from getting dry and irritated in the first place. By understanding how nature combats dryness in the winter to strengthen our immune system, we can begin to understand how to prevent colds and flu symptoms naturally. Making some simple seasonal shifts in the diet can make a huge difference in your child's health. Remember, if we were all still living on the farm, we would automatically reap the benefit of nature's medicine chest from each harvest. Most families are not too far off the mark. Most of us naturally crave more soups, grains, nuts, stews, and meats in the winter anyway! These are warm, insulating foods that help us combat the cold and dryness of winter. They are seasonal and harvested in the fall to be eaten in the winter.

Each Season Has Its Own Harvest and Suggested Meal Plan

In Chapter 7, you will find simple shopping lists with in-season foods to make eating with the seasons a no-brainer.

You should find your homework to be relatively easy. Simple things like knowing what season you are in and how to make certain food choices for your family will become some of your best medicinal techniques. If changing your family's diet is impossible, there are many other simple tips and supplementation ideas I will share to keep your kids healthy. You will learn how to assess your children's health and stress levels every morning. I have a Lazy Susan full of different herbs and supplements that I choose from daily according to each child's individual needs. You will learn how to recognize and then prevent a cold days in advance just by strengthening your child's digestion. I will teach you how to set up your own Lazy Susan and how to take the guesswork out of cold prevention.

More Homework

What situations make your kids more vulnerable to getting a cold? Are they eating too much candy? Are they eating their lunch at school? During those first days back to school, when the weather is getting colder and drier, your child will have a greater risk of catching a cold. Coming back from vacations, particularly after having traveled on airplanes or having gone to pool parties, will make your kids more susceptible to catching a cold. Mouth breathing while sleeping will dry the sinuses and potentially irritate mucous membranes, compromising immunity. I will explain in Chapter 9 simple things you can do during the times of heightened vulnerability to colds and flus to keep the runny nose running the other way. Once you evaluate your children with regard to these factors, it will become obvious what you need to do to take them out of cold's way.

Nutritional supplementation is another important area for health maintenance and disease prevention. And it is not as simple as just popping a morning vitamin pill. There are better times of year to take particular vitamins. We are used to thinking of RDA values as a reference for daily intake; after all, they are named the Recommended *Daily* (now called *Dietary*) Allowance. But nature's cycle of vitamin supplementation is annual, not daily.

With each changing season animals stay healthy by changing the amounts of vitamins, nutrients, and minerals they ingest from a naturally harvested diet that changes from one season to the next. In a world where everyone is trying to sell you and your family supplements, I have found it important for my patients and family to have a framework for understanding when and why to use supplements. Just as foods are harvested in certain seasons for the benefit of our health, herbal medicines also have a similar logic for their seasonal harvest.

Probably the most common example of this is the pesky dandelion weed. There is a reason why this weed is abundant in the spring and fall, and you'll find a similar logic for all plants. Allergies are a common cause of colds in the spring and fall. Dandelions have natural diuretic and blood-purifying properties and beneficial effects on the reduction of allergies and the prevention of colds. I am not pushing dandelions here, but it should be stated that 100 years ago, dandelion tea was a staple of the American diet. Bitter roots and veggies like dandelions, kale, swiss chard, and burdock root, all harvested in the spring and fall, were all part of the American diet, though today they are conspicuously missing from average American meals. I don't expect your kids to savor the flavor of swiss chard or spend afternoons munching on dandelions in the backyard, but there are ways to get the benefits of these bitter foods by hiding them in soups or through supplementation.

If you choose supplements, it is important to know when to use them, which are the best for your child in each season, and why. Remember, a large proportion of your immune-building minerals and vitamins comes from fruits and vegetables. If you doubt the nutritional power of fruits and veggies, look at an elephant, an elk, or a moose. They are huge, with impressive, vegetarian-made tusks and antlers. Because we eat meat in addition to vegetables, it

> In nature, animals do not get all their nutritional needs met on a daily basis as our RDA suggests. They have, as we do, a nutritional cycle that takes a year to complete.

should not be a problem for us to obtain the necessary nutrition to support a healthy immune system.

How Is Your Child's Digestion?

For years, the number one ailment I have treated in my practice has been constipation. Many of us are not even aware that we are constipated. Kids in particular do not think much about the last time they had a bowel movement. I don't think I've met a child in my practice yet who could remember exactly when he or she went to the bathroom in the past two days. Sadly, parents are seldom aware of the eliminative patterns of their children. It is very common for me to discover that a child who has chronic asthma and colds is also chronically and quietly constipated. Some of these kids go to the toilet only every other day and think nothing of it. Others commonly go two or three days without having a bowel movement with no immediately noticeable problems. Then their parents bring them into my office with chronic skin problems, colds, allergies, or breathing difficulties.

Few parents realize that there might be a connection between their child's poor health and sluggish bowel habits. Begin to watch and ask questions. I am sure most holistic doctors would agree that childhood constipation is a common cause of many health concerns that now face adults. In Chapter 4, I will explain how to prevent and treat constipation and how it can cause colds along with a host of other ailments.

Perfect Health

Ayurveda gives us many not-so-secret methods to improve the body's ability to take care of itself. I will describe many time- tested herbal therapies that have proved invaluable for keeping kids healthy. These herbs are all safe for children and are an incredibly valuable part of the plan for achieving and maintaining perfect health. The goal is not to create a dependency on herbs or supplements for any condition, rather to use herbs or other substances to strengthen the body and then allow children to stop taking the herb as quickly as possible.

So many kids are hooked on laxatives, digestive enzymes, inhalers, and antibiotics. If children become dependent on a pharmaceutical medication or even a medicinal herb early in life, they may end up taking it for years and endure side effects.

Using herbs to strengthen the body (rather than do something for the body) means that Ayurveda can work in combination with any pharmaceuticals or treatments your child is already taking or using. The two approaches can be complementary. There are times when a symptom must be dealt with. During these times, the body can simultaneously be made stronger so that the drug to suppress the symptoms can eventually be decreased and possibly even eliminated. In this book, my goal is not to contradict Western medicine, but to work closely with it.

You should always start with a Western doctor for accurate diagnosis, and to make sure you know the severity of the condition and whether you have ample time to explore natural therapies. Inform your primary care provider of your plan to use more natural forms of medicine. Often, Western medicine primary care providers will work in conjunction with an alternative or complementary provider to monitor a treatment plan. The information in this book is not intended to replace the diagnosis or treatment of your medical doctor or qualified health care practitioner. It is designed to be used in conjunction with your family doctor.

Ayurvedic Health Insurance

In the ancient, traditional beginnings of Ayurvedic medicine, Ayurvedic doctors were paid to keep the people under their care healthy. When someone fell ill, the doctor's pay was withheld until the person was well again. This does not mean that the doctor saw only unhealthy patients. On the contrary, doctors took an active role in providing their patients with the tools, herbs, dietary recommendations, and education to monitor and maintain their perfect health on a daily basis. In that same vein, this book is meant to provide parents with the tools from the era when the motivation of doctors was to keep their patients healthy. By understanding the ten ancient secrets of prevention and the means to address the causes of diseases

> Most of all, you will enjoy your family and children so much more when the fear of poor health is replaced with the gift of Perfect Health.

before they arise, parents can work in harmony with their doctors while becoming less and less dependent on them.

Simple Ayurvedic principles offer you and your children habits to ensure perfect health throughout your lives. As I watch my children grow up, I see that the tenets of good health are as ingrained as doing their own laundry. Teaching children how to take care of their own health is as important as teaching them how to make their own bed or cook their own meals.

Remember to implement the practices suggested in this book slowly. Test them out. Ayurvedic medicine is based on observation and cause and effect. These time-tested remedies will soon lead you to find that you prefer a more balanced lifestyle. At the first sniffle you will naturally reach for an herb rather than an over-the-counter cold medicine.

You don't have to be a believer in alternative medicine for these techniques to work. They will prove themselves. They have already been around for 5,000 years—plenty of time to discover and discard the therapies that were risky, dangerous, or just didn't work.

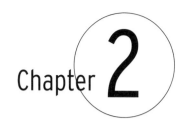

Chapter 2

Secret 1—Do You Know Who Your Kids Are?

Have you ever wondered why some kids get allergies and some don't? Why some tend to gain weight and others struggle to keep it on? Why some kids are interested in sports and others can't be bothered? Answers to these questions are described in many ancient medical systems, including Ayurveda.

If you take your car to a mechanic the first question you're asked is, "What is the model and year?" Similarly, we should ask, "What is the model of this child? Is she a Ford or a Chevy, or maybe a high-maintenance Porsche?" Knowing this information in the beginning can save you many headaches later on.

Every car comes with an owner's manual that tells you all the things you will need to do to keep the car in perfect running order. In the same way, the body and personality type of your children will give you, as a parent, the equivalent of an owner's manual: all the information you will need to maintain their mental, emotional, and physical balance for their entire lives. If the owner's manual and maintenance schedules are not followed, a car will drop in performance or develop problems just as a child will develop an imbalance. For example, just as the car may not start well in cold weather, children may develop breathing difficulties and asthma. Unfortunately, the owner's manual doesn't help when the car doesn't start. Likewise, the body type is most useful for keeping your child healthy, but only somewhat useful when your child is sick. Step one is to educate you about how to treat your children preventatively, when they are healthy. Knowing the body type of your child is a valuable tool.

In this chapter, I will introduce three basic body types that combine to give ten unique and different body types. One of these ten types will most accurately describe your child. I will describe the detailed owner's manual and list of maintenance requirements that correspond to each "kid type." It is important for parents to understand the individual nature of their children and follow these maintenance schedules to keep your children on the road to perfect health.

Each kid-type will be more or less susceptible to certain conditions, such as asthma or constipation, as well as behavior traits like shyness or anger. If a child develops an imbalance, treatments specific to the child's problem must be utilized. It is useful to know the body type of the child when treating for an imbalance in the same way it is important for a mechanic to know whether he or she is working on a Ford or a Chevy. It is also important that parents begin to educate their children, by example and lifestyle, about how to live in harmony with their individual body types so they can be prepared to carry their perfect health into adulthood.

> Traditional systems of medicine describe our connections to the graceful ebb and flow of nature's cycles. Ayurveda in particular studies and explains our relationship to nature. If we slow down for a moment and tune into our environment, it becomes obvious that we are intimately connected to these natural cycles. We are connected through our responses to nature's daily, weekly, monthly, and seasonal patterns.

Inner Rhythms

The way we respond to nature's cycles differs for each of us, and some of the more common personality traits are just variations in the way different body types cycle through the changes and natural rhythms of the day. Why are some people night owls while others are early birds? How many people feel an afternoon lull, but get a second wind at 10:00 P.M.? How many of us know someone who is cold all the time, or who can't stand the heat? We all know people who for no apparent reason hold onto more weight, are light sleepers, or have photographic memories. Stress is another part of the natural rhythm we all respond differently to: some of us tend toward depression while others tend toward anger. All these traits are budding in our children and the sooner we can become aware of them, the better we can protect their mental and physical health.

If we examine the changing cycles in nature, we find that the three basic kid-types seem to mirror these cycles. For example, the winter season is cold and dry—and there are people who naturally have a tendency for cold hands and feet and very dry skin. These are people we would describe as having a winter-like body type, since they express qualities that mirror the seasonal properties of winter. Summer is hot; correspondingly there are people who overheat more easily than others. These hot summer types who don't like the heat tend to contract more hot inflammatory conditions like heartburn or skin redness and rashes. In the spring when the rains come, the earth becomes muddy and congested. People who carry a lot of spring qualities hold onto water readily and tend to be heavier and more easy-going than the quick moving cold and dry winter types or the hot, fiery, and sharp summer types. Children are born with a certain amount of each of these three qualities, which translate into three basic body types—winter, summer, and spring. These three basic types combine with each other to form ten different and unique mind-body kid-types.

After studying many of the published body-type systems, I have found the Ayurvedic system to be the most useful for describing the whole person. It takes into consideration the mental, emotional, behavioral, and physical attributes of each individual. Most of the modern body-type systems are derivations of William Sheldon's Somatotyping work. He described three basic body types: the ectomorph, thin and frail like the winter body type in Ayurveda; the mesomorph, a medium-framed, muscular body type that relates to the summer type; and the endomorph, a bigger and heavier build that relates to spring. What seems to be missing in these typing systems—in a practical sense—is that people are not only physical in nature. We are also a complex matrix of body, mind, spirit, and emotions. Without understanding all of these factors, we may not really know why our children tick the way they do. The Ayurvedic typing system helps us to understand the whole child, which is an important first step to treating him or her successfully.

 Secret 1: The first health secret is for parents to understand exactly who their children are. Children are like fingerprints—no two are exactly alike. And children, like all of us, have different body types, personalities, and emotional make-ups. It is important for parents to help their children stay healthy by becoming tuned into the uniqueness of each child as early as possible.

The Three Types

In the Ayurvedic system, three basic types are described. The first, which depicts the winter season, is called Vata, or air. The second, reflected by summer, is called Pitta, or fire. The third, because of its tendency to hold water, reflects spring and is called Kapha, or earth and water.

To better understand these kid-types, visualize winter as cold, dry, windy, with the same qualities as the elements of air and space. Imagine summer as heat, having its source in the element of fire. And think of spring's heavy rains and mud that are wet like the elements of earth and water. The three basic kid-types—Vata = winter, Pitta = summer, and Kapha = spring—are made up of the five basic elements or building blocks of nature: space, air, fire, water, and earth.

The Three Doshas

The three doshas (Vata, Pitta, and Kapha) are the basic governing agents of the physiology. The doshas are made up of five fundamental elements found throughout nature: space, air, fire, water, and earth.

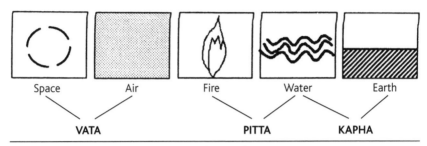

Fig. 1: 5 elements and relationship to the 3 kid-types

As you can see, winter, or Vata, is derived from a combination of air and space. In nature, cold and dry qualities are most dramatically expressed in the windy fall and winter. In the body, air is responsible for movement, including breathing, elimination, circulation, and the rapid firing of nerves.

Summer, or Pitta, is made of fire with a touch of water—to keep fire from burning the pot. Heat is expressed in nature most strongly in the summer months, and in the body is responsible for the functioning of the skin and liver, as well as the processes of digestion in the stomach and small intestine. Pitta controls vision and our competitive drive.

Spring, or Kapha, is a combination of earth and water. Because it is endowed with nature's heavy and solid elements, spring tends to have slow and methodical qualities. In the body, it is responsible for structural strength and stability, and maintaining an appropriate fluid balance. The interplay of these two innocent elements—earth and water—can cause us to come down with colds when they are out of balance. Remember, kids make mucus for a living. Anywhere you have mucus in the body, you have the wet qualities of spring brewing.

To summarize, Vata, Pitta, and Kapha reflect the three fundamental governing principles of nature: air and space, fire and water, and water and earth. At conception, each child is given some amount of each quality, and the proportion that the child has—the dominating qualities in the child's make-up—determines the his or her type. It is more than just a body type; it is a true psychophysiological, constitutional type or mind-body type. The Ayurvedic body type influences how a person thinks, spends money, eats, and sleeps, the size and shape of the body, and more. To simplify matters, I will describe each kid-type by season.

CHARACTERISTICS OF WINTER TYPE

- Light, thinner build
- Performs activity quickly
- Tendency toward dry skin
- Aversion to cold weather (feels cold easily)
- Irregular hunger and digestion
- Quick to grasp new information, also quick to forget
- Tendency toward worry
- Tendency toward constipation
- Tendency toward light and interrupted sleep

CHARACTERISTICS OF SUMMER TYPE

- Moderate build
- Performs activity with medium speed
- Aversion to hot weather (feels hot easily)
- Prefers cold food and drinks
- Sharp hunger and digestion
- Can't skip meals
- Medium time to grasp new information
- Medium memory
- Tendency toward reddish hair and complexion, moles, and freckles
- Good public speakers
- Tendency toward irritability and anger
- Enterprising and sharp in character

CHARACTERISTICS OF SPRING BODY TYPE

- Solid, heavier build
- Greater strength
- Greater endurance
- Slow and methodical in activity
- Oily, smooth skin
- Slow digestion, mild hunger
- Tranquil, steady personality
- Slow to grasp new information, slow to forget
- Slow to become excited or irritated
- Sleep is heavy and long
- Hair is plentiful, thick, and wavy

Who Are Those Guys?

Let's take a look at the three basic kid-types in the classroom:

Justin—The Spontaneous Winter Child

The first type—winter—is epitomized in a fifth grade boy named Justin. Compared to the other kids, Justin is a little on the skinny side and is proud of being quick minded and fast moving—even speedy. Because of Justin's restless nature, his teacher is constantly asking him to settle down and be quiet. Remember that the Ayurvedic term for the winter body type is Vata, which means air and movement. By nature, air is light and moves quickly, easily, and often, and this quality predominates in Justin's body type. He moves quickly, thinks quickly, and forgets quickly. He has a hard time focusing on one project for any length of time because his mind constantly leaps from one thing to another.

Of the three learning styles recognized by most educators, Justin learns best auditorily rather than visually or kinesthetically (through movement). He usually does well in school because our present educational system strongly favors this body type. Almost all the information is delivered verbally and Justin, though a little nervous or anxious at times, has a natural mental and physical quickness that ultimately proves to be his greatest asset.

At home, Justin is the one with dry, flaky skin and possibly even eczema (a dry skin condition). If his skin is dry, then his intestines might be too, making him susceptible to constipation that can go unnoticed for years, both because no one asks about bathroom habits and because kids don't know what is normal. If you have a child with a winter body type, questions about elimination have to be asked. Normal elimination for a winter kid-type is one bowel movement a day, first thing in the morning. In Chapter 4, I explain how to bring your child's bathroom routine back into balance without using habit-forming laxatives.

Justin may not be the best sleeper. He may wake up easily during the night and find himself in Mom and Dad's bed way too often. Because of his quick-minded temperament he will be a thinker, so it is important to take precautions to prevent him from thinking too much and becoming a worrier. Worry and stress can deplete Justin, making him fatigued, run-down, and unable to handle life's everyday stresses. Stress is significant in children's lives, often coming from other children. Kids, as any parent knows, can be ruthless, making the process of socialization and feeling liked and accepted a struggle for any child. The winter kid-type is a higher maintenance body type and these children should be carefully guided through the stressful childhood years. They are particularly sensitive and parents need to offer them an insulating cushion.

Jessica—The Fiery Summer Child

Justin's classmate, Jessica, is a fiery summer kid-type. She learns best visually and excels in schoolwork, particularly in math and other visually oriented subjects. Jessica is an extremely competitive girl who is quick to take command and lead the class if necessary. Her fiery mind tends to drive her body hard, and she is something of a perfectionist. This trait often makes her the best at whatever she chooses to do, but on the negative side, it can make her overly demanding of herself. If she doesn't win or come out on top it can really get her down. In the summer months, Jessica's face turns bright red when she gets overheated, which isn't hard for her to do since her body type carries heat by nature.

Jessica is a bit more physically and mentally durable than her quick-minded classmate Justin, but parents need to be aware of her weaknesses in order for her to maintain perfect health. Because she runs hot, she has a tendency to develop more skin rashes and acne than other types. This heat may also affect her emotionally and she may tend toward anger, bad sportsmanship, and bullying if not guided at a young age. She is a natural leader, but may not always be well liked, as she can put other children down in an effort to make herself feel more important. We all know children like this and parents should intervene here and support more balanced behavior.

Summer kid-types are constitutionally strong and at a young age they don't have too many health problems. If they do get out of balance, you may see skin rashes, acne, loose bowel movements, irrational and hostile behavior, and poor eyesight. As they get older, these kid-types will be more susceptible to heartburn, ulcers, allergies, prostate, blood, and inflammatory conditions.

Hank—The Steady Spring Child

The third basic type is accurately embodied in Justin and Jessica's classmate Hank. One of the bigger boys in the class, Hank is a spring kid-type. By nature he is slow to learn, but once he "gets it," he's got it for life. He is just the opposite of Justin, who takes in information quickly but can't remember it for very long. Hank learns best kinesthetically. The problem is that most of his classes are taught visually, using textbooks, videos, and blackboard examples; or verbally, with lectures and discussions. He excels in geometry and geography, which allow him to learn kinesthetically (from pictures and shapes). Hank is a late bloomer, and will command any field of activity as he matures.

Hank's demeanor is calm and tranquil; people like him and feel comfortable around him. He moves slowly and methodically with no wasted effort. In our fast-paced world, Hank runs the risk of being labeled "slow" because he is a methodical thinker, but he has just as much talent and ability as his classmates.

Because Hank naturally possesses more water and earth elements, he makes more mucus than the other kid-types. He will be prone to colds and coughs and his parents have to be careful of mucus-producing foods like Mac 'n' Cheese and pizza for dinner and cold milk and cereal for breakfast. For Hank, these foods are an invitation for colds, earaches, allergies, and asthma.

Vigilance on the part of Hank and his parents is particularly important in the springtime when his body is naturally making more mucus. Just as the earth flows with more water in the spring in the form of rain and mud, our bodies also hold onto more water. Hank, due to his nature, will easily become congested, making him more susceptible to mucus-related conditions.

Hank, if he is a pure spring kid-type, may be at risk of gaining weight. This can easily be avoided if his proclivities for eating and his slower metabolism are detected and prevented early. Exercise will be important for Hank, but it had best be fun or he will have no interest in it. Running track for the joy of running will not be his cup of tea. He's short on agility, but has great physical endurance and strength. He needs a reason to move—like hitting a baseball or running for a touchdown. Hank's natural strength will make him popular when choosing up sides for football, and he will probably bat clean-up on the baseball team.

 Parental Tip: Each kid-type is a reflection of a child who is predominantly one type. In nature, this rarely occurs. In fact, each child will always be a unique combination of all three kid-types. How much of each of the three qualities of winter, summer, and spring a child has will determine the kid-type. In the above examples, the descriptions were extreme because each child displayed 100% of their respective quality. Jessica's intensity and heat, for example, would typically be offset by some qualities of one of the other kid-types. These combinations will be explained in more detail later in this chapter.

VATA CONSTITUTION

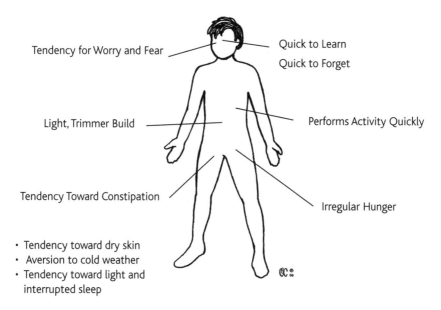

Tendency for Worry and Fear

Quick to Learn
Quick to Forget

Light, Trimmer Build

Performs Activity Quickly

Tendency Toward Constipation

Irregular Hunger

- Tendency toward dry skin
- Aversion to cold weather
- Tendency toward light and interrupted sleep

PITTA CONSTITUTION

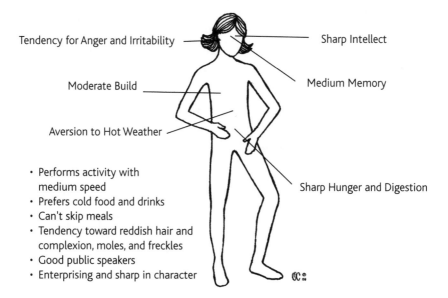

Tendency for Anger and Irritability

Sharp Intellect

Moderate Build

Medium Memory

Aversion to Hot Weather

- Performs activity with medium speed
- Prefers cold food and drinks
- Can't skip meals
- Tendency toward reddish hair and complexion, moles, and freckles
- Good public speakers
- Enterprising and sharp in character

Sharp Hunger and Digestion

KAPHA CONSTITUTION

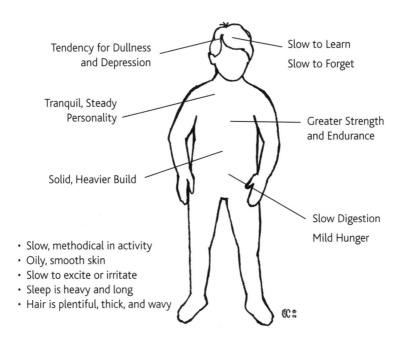

Tendency for Dullness and Depression

Slow to Learn

Slow to Forget

Tranquil, Steady Personality

Greater Strength and Endurance

Solid, Heavier Build

Slow Digestion

Mild Hunger

- Slow, methodical in activity
- Oily, smooth skin
- Slow to excite or irritate
- Sleep is heavy and long
- Hair is plentiful, thick, and wavy

A Delicate Balance

As we can see from the stories of Justin, Jessica, and Hank, each child has a unique make up. The kid-types should seem familiar as we have all seen aspects of these three examples in our own children and in their friends. But knowing your children's kid-types does more than just tell you who they are and what they are good at; one of the fringe benefits of knowing your children's kid-types is recognizing the difference between balanced and unbalanced behavior.

 Parental Tip: By knowing what traits make your children who they are, you can identify behaviors they exhibit when they are out of balance. Once you become familiar with the normal traits of your child's kid-type, then the abnormal or unbalanced ones will be obvious and treatable days or weeks before more severe symptoms arise.

When a child is in balance, this does not mean that the properties of winter, summer, and spring are exactly equal. It simply means that the body type is functioning in harmony with both its external and internal environments. Balance in the body promotes healthy physical, mental, and emotional function. The following is a basic guideline for balanced and unbalanced physical traits and behaviors of each kid-type.

Balanced winter kid-types reflect:

- Mental alertness
- Grace and coordination
- Creativity and artistic ability
- Articulate speech
- Slender frame
- Proper formation of body tissues
- Normal elimination
- Sound sleep
- Strong immunity
- Sense of exhilaration

Imbalance in winter kid-types creates:

- Dry or rough skin
- Insomnia
- Constipation
- Fatigue
- Headaches
- Intolerance of cold
- Underweight or loss of weight
- Anxiety, worry and restlessness
- Attention deficit with hyperactivity

Balanced summer kid-types reflect:

- Warm body temperature
- Normal thirst mechanisms
- Strong digestion

- Lustrous complexion
- Sharp intellect
- Intense drive and motivation
- Healthy competitive edge
- Natural leadership abilities
- Contentment

Imbalance in summer kid-types creates:

- Rashes
- Inflammatory skin conditions (including acne)
- Stomachaches
- Diarrhea
- Controlling and manipulative behavior
- Visual problems or burning in the eyes
- Excessive body heat
- Hostility, irritability
- Excessive competition

Balanced spring kid-types reflect:

- Muscular strength
- Vitality and stamina
- Strong immunity
- Affection, generosity, courage, dignity
- Stability of mind
- Healthy, normal joints
- Great memory
- Thick, strong hair and nails

> When the body drifts out of balance, the harmony of mind and body is lost and the beginning signs and symptoms of imbalance are seen.

Imbalance in spring kid-types creates:

- Oily skin
- Slow or sluggish digestion
- Sinus congestion
- Nasal allergies
- Asthma

- Obesity
- Skin growths
- Possessiveness, neediness
- Apathy
- Depression
- Spaceyness
- Difficulty paying attention

Kid-Type Assessment Tool

There are five profiles in this assessment that will be interpreted to gain deeper insight into the whole child. These are the mental, behavioral, emotional, physical, and fitness profiles. Some children may have a very strong mental profile with high intelligence but may be less strong emotionally, which may contribute to a rockier road developmentally. Having this information helps parents support their children and understand their developmental challenges.

Instructions

When completing these profiles for your child, it may not be possible to respond to each category accurately. As your child grows, you will be able to choose responses at an age-appropriate time. If your child does not fit any of the three possible categories, then just leave the row blank. On the other hand, if your child really fits into all three, or two of three, then circle all that apply. Remember, however, the goal of the assessment is to find the dominant traits of your child. If your child has some tendency to one of the answers but strongly identifies with another, then only choose the one that really stands out, leaving the others blank.

It may be helpful for parents to first answer the questions for the child, depending on the child's age. Some of these questions may benefit from discussion between parents and their child. Sometimes the most accurate results come from a combination of the input from parents and child.

When you are finished, tally each section, then add the five profile subtotals to determine your child's kid-type.

Note: If this is a library book, please be kind to future readers and keep your score on a separate piece of paper or write lightly in pencil.

MENTAL PROFILE

	WINTER	SUMMER	SPRING
Mental activity	Quick mind, restless ✓	Sharp intellect agressive	Calm, steady, stable
Memory	Short-term best ✓	Good overall	Long-term best
Thoughts	Always changing ✓	Generally steady	Steady, stable, fixed
Concentration	Short-term best ✓	Better than average	Good ability for long-term focus
Ability to learn	Quick grasp ✓	Medium grasp	Slow grasp
Dreams	Fearful, flying, running, jumping, ✓	Angry fiery, violent, adventurous	Include water, clouds, relationships, love
Sleep	Interrupted, light ✓	Sound, medium	Sound, heavy, long
Voice	High pitch	Medium pitch ✓	Low pitch
Mental Subtotal	(7)	\	

BEHAVIORAL PROFILE

	WINTER	SUMMER	SPRING
Eating speed	Quick	Medium	Slow ✓
Hunger level	Irregular ✓	Sharp, needs food when hungry	Can easily miss meals
Food and drink	Prefers warm	Prefers cold ✓	Prefers dry and warm
Achieving goals	Easily distracted	Focused and dedicated ✓	Slow and steady
Sharing and giving	Gives a little	Large, infrequent giving ✓	Gives generously
Works best	While supervised	Alone ✓	In groups
Weather preference	Aversion to cold	Aversion to heat ✓	Aversion to damp, cold
Reaction to stress	Excites quickly ✓	Medium	Slow to get excited
Piggy bank	Doesn't save, spends quickly ✓	Saves, but big spender	Saves regularly accumulates wealth
Friendships	Makes friends easily short-term friends	Tends to be a loner friends often related	Tends to form long-lasting friendships ✓
Behavioral Subtotal	3	(5)	2

EMOTIONAL PROFILE

	WINTER	SUMMER	SPRING
Moods	Changes quickly ✓	Changes slowly	Steady, unchanging
Reacts to stress with	Fear ✓	Anger memory ✓	Indifference
Sensitive to	Own feelings ✓	Not sensitive	Others' feelings
If threatened, tends to	Run	Fight ✓	Make peace
Relations with parents	Clingy	Jealous ✓	Secure
Expresses Affection	With words	With actions	With touch ✓
When feeling hurt	Cries	Argues ✓	Withdraws
Emotional trauma causes	Anxiety ✓	Anger ✓	Depression
Confidence level	Timid	Outwardly self-confident ✓	Inner confidence
Emotional Subtotal	4	⑥	1

PHYSICAL PROFILE

	WINTER	SUMMER	SPRING
Amount of hair	Thin	Average ✓	Thick
Hair type	Dry	Normal ✓	Oily
Hair color	Light brown, blonde ✓	Red, auburn	Dark brown, black
Skin	Dry, rough ✓	Soft, medium	Oily, moist, cool
Skin temperature	Cold hands/feet	Warm ✓	Cool
Complexion	Darker	Pink-red ✓	Pale-white
Eyes	Small	Medium ✓	Large
Whites of eyes	Blue/brown	Yellow/red	White/glossy
Size of teeth	Very large or very small	Small-medium ✓	Medium-large
Weight	Thin, hard to gain	Medium ✓	Heavy, gains easily
Elimination	Dry, hard, thin ✓ easily constipated	Many during day, soft to normal	Heavy, slow, thick, regular
Physical Subtotal	3	⑦	

FITNESS PROFILE

	WINTER	SUMMER	SPRING
Exercise tolerance	Low ✓	Medium	High
Endurance	Fair ✓	Good	Excellent
Strength	Fair	Good ✓	Excellent
Speed	Very good	Good ✓	Not so fast
Competition	Doesn't like ✓ pressure to compete	Driven, competitive	Deals easily with pressure to compete
Walking speed	Fast ✓	Average	Slow and steady
Muscle tone	Slim	Average ✓	Brawny
Runs like	Deer	Tiger ✓	Bear
Body size	Small frame, lean or long	Medium frame ✓	Large frame, fleshy
Reaction time	Quick	Average	Slow ✓
Fitness Subtotal	4	(5)	1

TOTALS

	WINTER	SUMMER	SPRING
Mental	7	1	
Behavioral	3	5	2
Emotional	4	6	1
Physical	3	7	
Fitness	4	5	1
Kid-Type	21	24	4

Pitta-Vatta

How To Use This Information

Tallying the five constitutional profiles will allow you to see your child's traits and behavioral patterns divided into the three kid-type categories. As every child has at least a little of each of the three constitutional principles—winter, summer, and spring—the scores are seldom perfectly clear-cut. Due to the variations of possible results, the three basic kid-types are divided into ten possible proportional combinations. The body type will help reveal your child's potential weak links, giving you insight into ways of supporting and protecting your child's well-being.

Look at the total scores to determine your child's kid-type. For example, if the totals read: 26 Winter, 15 Summer, and 11 Spring, then the child expresses high winter properties and we call this child a winter kid-type. This means the child will tend to exhibit the qualities of winter, such as being light, cold, fast, and restless. This child may be more susceptible to feeling chilly, becoming dried out, and catching a cold in the winter.

If the score is: 15 Winter, 26 Summer, and 11 Spring, then this child is a summer kid-type. The child will tend to have a medium frame with a driven and competitive nature. If the natural drive and heat in this kid-type are not understood, then they can easily burn out and develop heat- and stress-related health problems.

If the score is: 9 Winter, 15 Summer, and 26 Spring, then this child is a spring kid-type. The child will likely have a larger frame and an easy-going personality. He or she will be more susceptible to colds, asthma, and flus, particularly in the spring. I will describe preventive techniques designed to support your child in times of stress and high cold risk.

If the score is: 18 Winter, 21 Summer, and 19 Spring, then the child has a constitution with a nearly equal amount of all three seasonal attributes—a Tri-Type. As a result, the child's constitution will be strong. But these tri-types must be careful. They need to be preventively minded in each season because they carry an abundant quantity of each principle. In the winter, if they do not eat enough warm and high-fat foods, they will dry out and freeze. In the summer they will be equally susceptible to the heat, and in the spring, the moisture. This is a high-performance race car with a constant maintenance schedule.

In analyzing the profile results, it may be most common to find that two of the principles predominate, and the constitution or kid-type is a combination of two principles. In this case you might tally: 25 Winter, 23 Summer, and 8 Spring. The winter and summer properties are nearly equal with a low spring tally. We call this child a winter-summer kid-type. If the score is skewed to be more summer than winter—let's say: 21 Winter, 26 Summer, 15 Spring—then the child is a summer-winter kid-type. The three basic types can combine to make ten unique kid-types are:

- Winter
- Summer
- Spring
- Winter-Summer
- Winter-Spring
- Summer-Winter
- Summer-Spring
- Spring-Winter
- Spring-Summer
- Winter-Summer-Spring or Tri-Type

When someone is a combination of two kid-types, like a winter-summer or winter-spring, the qualities of both seasons will be present. It is conventional to write the predominant quality first. The one written second will be a strong influence in the kid-type, but not as strong as the first.

Using the Profiles

To understand exactly how these qualities make up the personality and behavioral traits of your child, you can look individually at the scores of each of the five profiles: mental, behavioral, emotional, physical, and fitness.

Knowing the kid-types gives you a distinct advantage in keeping your children healthy. Throughout this book I will provide an interpretation of what this information means. But there is more insight to be gained from the body type profiles than just understanding a child's body type. The breakdown of the five profiles gives specific information about how kid-types express themselves in different facets of a child's body and personality. We can discover a great deal more detail about children's traits by looking at the subtotals of each profile.

Sally's Overall Profile
Winter 10, Summer 21, Spring 19
Summer-Spring Kid-Type
Sally. is a summer-spring kid-type with strong and nearly equal amounts of both summer and spring.
The breakdown of the five profiles will identify which traits of summer and spring are inherently expressed.

Sally's Mental Profile
Winter 10, Summer 12, Spring 26
Spring Mental Type
Sally's mental profile is a variation from her kid-type score. Even though Sally may be an overall summer-spring kid-type, she thinks like a pure spring kid-type. This may explain Sally's thoughtful, slow, and methodical nature and why she may not be the speediest reader or best test-taker. Since Sally is generally influenced by the fiery and intense qualities of summer, it is reasonable to presume that as she gets older she will grow out of these slow springlike mental qualities. In Chapter 3, I will describe the three phases of a human life. The first phase is the spring phase, which make spring qualities more noticeable in a child who often later outgrows them.

Randy's Overall Profile
Winter 25, Summer 14, Spring 9
Winter Kid-type
Randy's tally describes a winter kid-type who will display predominately winter-like behavior.

If you scan Randy's profile subtotals, winter does not have the highest score in each one. This will help to explain why all of Randy's behaviors do not fit exactly into any one of the kid-types. He has higher winter scores except in the fitness profile.

Randy's Fitness Profile
Winter 15, Summer 25, Spring 23
Summer-Spring Fitness Type
These scores tell us that even though Randy is a winter kid-type with a quick and delicate nervous system, from a fitness point of view he will perform well with greater strength and stamina than the final total would suggest.

How This Information Can Be Useful

Let's say that your child is having difficulty in physical education, or that his or her reading comprehension is lower than grade level, or he or she is shy or even bossy. If you carefully review each profile looking for a category that doesn't match the final kid-type tally, you will likely discover important insights into your child's strengths and weaknesses. For example, a child who is a summer-spring overall kid-type may have a predominantly winter mental profile. This could explain why this child is anxious and worries easily, even though their overall profile would indicate otherwise. This information gives you a map to understand your child's traits and help offset any extreme tendencies.

Body Types to the Rescue

In 1960, East Germany started body-typing their young children to help improve their Olympic success. They used a variety of body-typing parameters that yielded great results for a country the size of

New York State. In 1968, East Germany won nine gold medals and the U.S. won 45. In 1976, East Germany won 47 gold medals and the U.S. won 37. I am not suggesting that we use body-type information in this way; rather I'm acknowledging that many behavioral and physical traits are apparent at a very young age. For parents, this information can be helpful for preventing and treating the ailments a child is susceptible to, it can explain personality and teenage behavior, and it can assist in choosing exercise and fitness activities that allow a child to excel.

Unfortunately, many kids experience emotional trauma in gym class. Frequently, coaches and P.E. teachers require children to climb the ropes successfully or run a mile in under ten minutes to receive a passing grade. Every child is different, and not all are going to be able to perform at this level. In fact, when they cannot climb the ropes or run a mile in under ten minutes, or when they're the last child picked for the softball or soccer team, they experience public humiliation—an experience that discouraged many small lives from doing any sports and fitness, which is ultimately damaging to their health. In one Louis Harris Poll, it was reported that "50% of all American kids experience their first major failure in life as a sports failure."

Knowing Who Your Children Are

This poll was what I had in mind when I visited a private school on the west coast to talk to coaches about body-types and how to avoid some of the emotional trauma kids endure in gym class. Understanding a child's kid-type can change lives, the way it did with young Sharon. Sharon knew why I was visiting her school and came up to me right after her gym class. She was about 10 years old, and had just finished struggling around the track in a test for the one-mile run. Her beautiful, round face was beet red, and sweat was still dripping off her nose. She was totally exhausted, discouraged, and dejected.

"Dr. Douillard," she said, "can you write me an excuse to get out of gym class?"

"Don't you like gym?" I asked her.

"I hate it."

"Why? Isn't it fun?"

"It's no fun at all."

"Isn't there anything about it that you like?"

"No," Sharon said, "I'm not good at anything." Sharon was a Babe Ruth, spring kid-type with a solid frame and bone structure. Although speed was not Sharon's strong suit, with her natural strength, endurance, and coordination, there were many sports she could excel in and enjoy.

As she continued to tell me what happened on the track, she began to cry. "Everyone was running as fast as they could," she said. "The coaches were yelling at us and blowing their whistles, telling us to go faster. I was hurting so bad, and trying as hard as I could, but I just couldn't go any faster. I finished in 11 minutes and 30 seconds."

I knew that in order to get a passing grade, the kids had to run the mile in 10 minutes. I knew that was a tall order for Sharon's age and kid-type. Sharon is not the only one—50% of American school girls can't run a mile in 10 minutes.

"It's just not fair," she said, wiping the tears off her cheeks. "I tried my very best." And then she added the clincher: "And all the other kids were watching. and I was the last one. "

My heart went out to her. I knew she was sincere and that the kind of exercise she was being asked to do would likely make her hate exercise for the rest of her life. Right there in front of her fourth grade she was turning into one of the 85% of adult Americans who don't exercise. I knew I couldn't write her a note, so I went to talk to her P.E. teacher.

It was clear that if Sharon were to keep getting tested and graded as a runner, several things would happen. First, she would fail the class. Second, she would feel humiliated by the experience. Third, she would reject exercise entirely, and probably become drastically out of shape, even while she's a child. Fourth, her childhood humiliation and failure would stay with her into her adult life and contribute to how she will accept challenges. The childhood years are the "wonder years"—a time when we must feed our kids with the proper physical, mental, and emotional nutrition, otherwise problems will surely surface later on. All that's necessary to keep children like Sharon from having to endure this worst-case but not farfetched scenario is to help them discover the kind of exercise that suits their body type and makes them happy.

Luckily, Sharon's P.E. teacher was open-minded and understood the antiquated nature of the President's Council on Physical Fitness test. He was open to learning how to determine body-types and how to select a wide range of exercise programs.

His vision gives this story a happy ending. About a year later, I received a phone call from Sharon's mother. She told me—with some amazement and a great deal of pride—that Sharon was going to compete in the regional championships as a race walker. Out of self-protection, Sharon had previously defined herself as a bookworm and was fully prepared to sacrifice the development of her body for the sole development of her mind. Finding a sport she enjoyed and could succeed rekindled her interest in sports. Her mother was thrilled that she was exploring new territory and becoming a more well-rounded person—maybe even an athlete.

The next time I visited Sharon's school, she told me excitedly about her race-walk competition and how her favorite class in school was now P.E. She also told me with great enthusiasm that she had just joined the basketball team. I was thrilled and speechless. She said, "The little body-types dribble the ball around while I get rebounds." She was so proud of her new-found, self-esteem building, athletic self-image as a "rebounder." It was hard for me to believe that this was the same little girl who a year earlier had begged me in tears for a note to permanently excuse her from P.E. It is easy to see how close Sharon came to missing the mental, physical, and emotional health benefits of exercise.

 Note: Parts of Sharon's story were excerpted from my book, *Body, Mind, and Sport.*

Sharon was not the first child to approach me and ask for help in getting out of P.E. As parents, we can use the kid-type information and profile scores to help prevent these sports failures by directing our children into something they will excel at and enjoy. By encouraging them to pursue activities appropriate for who they are, we can feed children with the passion for play—an essential nutrient for children of all ages.

Parental Tip: Use your knowledge of your children's kid-types to encourage them to choose physical activities and sports which they will enjoy. By helping them choose activities they can excel at, you will start them on the road to exercise, movement, and play, which they will then walk down the rest of their lives.

Play is only one of life's essential nutrients, and I will describe play in further detail in Chapters 11 and 12. Understanding your children's kid-types can help you find ways to provide them with the proper nutrients for all parts of their lives. As we move into the next chapters, we will see how each kid-type presents different health susceptibilities and concerns. We often need to treat children of different kid-types a little differently—simply due to their unique constitutional make-up. The first step to keeping your kids healthy is knowing who your children are and why it is they do what they do.

Chapter 3

Secret 2—Kids Make Mucus for a Living

Mucus is something we don't usually discuss in polite conversation. But as a parent, it is a part of your daily life, because kids make a lot of mucus. It seems like kids always need to wipe or blow their noses. Though it can seem like a nuisance, especially since kids frequently have runny noses and coughs, mucus production is an extremely important part of being a kid. In fact, it's an important part of being a person.

Mucus production is an important part of the body's lubrication and immunity. For kids, this lubrication is extremely significant because it supports their elastic growth—up to a foot each year. The amount of lubrication in a kid's body is one reason why a 7-year-old child can slide down a set of stairs laughing with each bump whereas an 80-year-old would simply break.

Sometimes the body produces excessive amounts of mucus as a result of drying out. When our sinuses get dry, they get irritated, and we react by making more mucus in an attempt to increase lubrication. This reactive mucus can overshoot the body's requirements and become too much of a good thing as it clogs up sinuses and mucous membranes, leading to congestion and providing a breeding ground for infectious bacteria and other microorganisms.

The immune system uses the mucous membranes as first line of defense for fighting infections. The exact amount of mucus production is crucial. Just like the story of Goldilocks and the Three Bears, it has to be *just right,* not too much mucus and not too little. Different kid-types have natural tendencies toward different amounts of dryness or of mucus production in the body. These different tendencies lead to varying levels of susceptibility to things like colds, flu, asthma, or other respiratory conditions. Another factor that affects each kid-type differently is the movement of the seasonal influences through the cycles of a person's life. In kids, mucus production is especially heavy during their first 12 years. Once a child reaches the teenage years, mucus production usually slows down or stops altogether, at which time we we often see childhood asthma conditions spontaneously get better. Mucus production is usually fairly stable during the middle years of life. Then as we move into our senior years we being to dry out, making less mucus and other lubricants.

The Human Lifecycle

Spring

In nature, spring is a time of new growth, when everything starts up after a long winter's rest, just as childhood is the time of growth and beginnings in the human lifecycle. In nature, the lubricating rains come in the spring, and in the same way, kids make lubricating mucus for a living. Rain supports the growth of new leaves, grass, and flowers just as mucus supports the rapid and elastic growth of children. In the same way a plant needs a moist environment to germinate and grow, children also require a moist medium. Children in the natural springtime of their lives who are also spring kid-types, run the risk of making excessive mucus, which can cause them to develop more colds and breathing difficulties than average.

Summer

All children grow out of the springtime cycle of their life at around age 12. They then move into the next season in the cycle—summer. In nature, summer is a very hot and active time of year. Plants and animals are much more active in the summer, taking advantage of the long days before the cold of winter sets in. If you were a bird, you would have to maximize your summer opportunity to learn to fly and feed yourself and then grow strong enough to travel thousands of miles to survive the coming winter. This is the nature of summer—intense and without a dull moment.

From the teenage years into our 50s is the most active time of our lives. It is the time when we are ready to take on the world, raise our children, and make our mark on society. A summer-type person may easily become overheated or be susceptible to a variety of inflammatory conditions. Adult summer-types are more susceptible to heartburn, heat and skin rashes, vision problems, arthritis, allergies, and blood disorders. Humans go through the summer cycle of life starting at age 12 and continue to the age of 50 or 60 when the winter cycle begins to set in.

Winter

Winter is the last season of the human lifecycle. In nature, winter is time of dormancy when animals hibernate or burrow underground, trees lose their leaves, and other plants quietly die back while their roots or seeds wait for the spring. This is a time of rest, when nature prepares itself to start over in the spring.

Just as the leaves dry and fall off the trees, we too dry out. Our skin becomes dry, and our joints lose their lubrication and become stiff. The body is winding down, but the mind is typically as sharp as ever. During this time of life, two major events begin to take place. The first is that the body begins to break down through a long drawn-out drying process. As we age and endure life stresses the muscles grow tighter, the body becomes stiffer and flexibility wanes. As a result, the ability of the blood supply to penetrate the deep tissues is slowly compromised. Without adequate blood supply, lubrication for the muscles, joints and organs is lost. More importantly, tissues are deprived of the oxygen carried by the blood. Without oxygen, the cells and tissues cannot survive. Inadequate oxygen can cause the body to lay down an abundance of fibrous scar tissue that requires very little blood supply, rendering the body stiff, brittle, and rigid. Hence, the aging process begins.

The second major event that takes place during the winter lifecycle is a growing spiritual inclination. In the winter lifecycle, the mind becomes more active and the body becomes less active. As winter, or Vata, reflects the qualities of air and lightness, the mind naturally drifts toward a more subtle and spiritual purpose.

> According to Ayurveda, spring is the heavy time of year relating to the structural parts of our body. Summer is hot and stimulating and is connected to the digestive system. Wintertime is cold and dry—so cold and dry, that even the water freezes and blows as snow. Winter represents movement in the body, controlling the nervous system and the mind.

The Grandparent Connection

Ayurveda, being a system of medicine that is 5,000 years old, has always depended on the wisdom of the elders to carry knowledge and pass it down to the next generation. Their wisdom and life experience were respected and revered. It is unfortunate that in our society we have lost respect for the wisdom of our elders. This is a loss that results in every generation starting anew. The terms "grand"mother and "grand"father signify having arrived at a place in life where one will live out their lives rich with wisdom, family, and grandeur.

The opportunity to have a close relationship with a grandparent not only enriches the childhood experience but has a significant effect on academic achievement. A study published in *Sociological Spectrum* in 1996 measured grade-point averages in multiple-generation families with children, parents, and grandparents living in the same home. High school grade point averages were higher—as were college aspirations—in multiple-generation families than they were in families without grandparents.

Sadly, it is more common today to isolate grandparents from the family and grandchildren. Children miss out on the mentorship of a grandparent, as well as the sense of security, guidance, and attention that having an extended family at home provides. This cannot be replaced with caregivers and after-school programs. If possible, when rearing a family, include grandparents as much as you can into the lives of your children. Although it is no longer customary to invite grandparents to live in an extended family arrangement, living close to grandparents should be seriously considered if possible. It benefits the grandchildren mentally, spiritually, and emotionally beyond measure.

> An important part of the path to maintaining good health is to know when you are susceptible to certain imbalances. If you're a spring-type in the spring lifecycle or a summer-type in the summer lifecycle, you are in a high-risk cycle. During these times it is important to follow the rules of your constitution more closely. Understanding these lifecycles, particularly for children under 12, is a key ingredient to perfect health for kids.

Secret 2: The second secret involves learning how to manage your children's tendency to make mucus. Kids under 12 are in the spring cycle of their lives where the production of mucus supports their rapidly growing bodies. While just the right amount of mucus is necessary, too much can lead to colds, plugged noses, and infections.

Not All Kids Make Mucus Equally

Our bodies are always trying to produce the right amount of mucus. The goal is to maintain a perfect balance in the mucous membranes that is not too dry or too wet. When balanced, mucus naturally moves throughout the body, over the mucous membranes and the lining of the sinuses. As the mucus moves, it carries bacteria, viruses, and other contaminants out with it. In our lungs, the thin coating of mobile mucus helps to protect us from the constant onslaught of environmental microbes and irritants. When mucus is excessive or becomes thick and stagnant inside the sinuses and other passageways, it becomes the perfect breeding ground for an infection.

For this reason, a typical American kid who eats lots of mucus-forming Mac 'n' Cheese, pizza, and fast foods has an increased chance of getting a cold. There is no doubt that kids get more colds, coughs, and earaches than adults, and it is all about those mucous membranes.When they dry out, the child may experience the first signs of a sore or scratchy throat. If this irritation lingers, the mucous membranes will produce excessive reactive mucus.

As I discussed in Chapter 2, each child is unique with different strengths, talents, likes, and dislikes, as well as health-related susceptibilities. An important health care guideline is to know who your child is, including his or her kid-type—with its strengths and weaknesses. Each kid-type does not make mucus in the same way or in the same amount.

Parental Tip: If your children are spring kid-types in the spring lifecycle (which they are if their under 12), it's important not to feed them foods which will aggravate their proclivity to make mucus, especially in the spring months. Reduce cold foods and drinks. cheese, ice cream, milkshakes, cold cereal and cold milk, ice water and ice drinks, Mac 'n' Cheese, and pizza. All these foods will be worse if eaten at night. (A complete list of appropriate seasonal foods is in Chapter 7.)

Spring Rains

Spring, or Kapha, kid-types will tend to be more like the spring rains, making more mucus and becoming more congested. Remember the spring kid-types are the bigger, heavier set kid-types with a slow and steady metabolism and nervous system. In spring, the earth holds more water, and it is the time of year that we typically get lots of rain and humidity. This is "allergy season." The spring kid-type will naturally produce more mucus than a dry winter kid-type. Of course, this can be compounded if the spring kid-type is eating an abundance of mucus-aggravating foods like fast food, deep-fried foods, and dairy products including: milk, ice cream, cheese, and pizza. If your spring kid-type eats this kind of diet during the spring months, you end up with a mucus-making kid in the mucus season eating mucus-producing foods: a cold, flu, or asthma attack just waiting to happen.

> Once you realize these simple and obvious facts, prevention of colds, allergies, and breathing difficulties will make sense and be effortless.

Breathing Freely

Many spring kid-types produce excessive mucus that obstructs the bronchioles, causing them breathing problems. At the first sign of wheezing, many parents bring their child to the doctor, who hangs the gloomy diagnosis of asthma over the child's head. The only hope offered is that the child may grow out of it as a teenager. But if not, the parents are told it is very possible that their child may fight asthma for the rest of his or her life.

According to a 1997 report by the Consumer Federation of America, asthma was once a relatively rare disease. Now the condition is extremely common—the national asthma rate has tripled in the last 20 years. Nearly 30 million Americans are currently afflicted. Childhood asthma has also increased. In fact, since 1980 the overall incidence of asthma has increased by more than 40%. According to the National Center for Health Statistics, as of 1997, the average child had visited the doctor 23 times during the first four years of life, most commonly for respiratory ailments. Diet, toxicity in the home, stress, and lack of exercise are just some of the causes of respiratory disease that I will address in the coming chapters.

Doctors prescribe inhalers or bronchodilators for wheezing children, and they work like magic. Within minutes, or even seconds, the airway is open and the child is breathing again. We are fortunate because these inhalers save lives and without them asthma would be a much more serious and life-threatening condition. But a problem with inhalers is that they can slowly stop working, leading to the need for an increased dosage, frequency of use, and then a stronger medication. This can happen because they are prescribed solely for relief of symptoms without attention to what may be the underlying cause. The inhaler dilates the bronchioles, but at the same time it irritates those very sensitive mucous membranes. When the mucous membranes get irritated, they produce reactive mucus. This increased mucus production can block the bronchioles, once again causing the breathing to become labored and requiring yet another dose of the inhaler—setting the cycle up once again. Additionally, the reactive mucus production increases the risk of establishing a fertile breeding ground for viral or bacterial infections. Once the wheezing starts, the child hits the inhaler. Relief is instant but the diagnosis of chronic asthma becomes a more permanent reality.

This story is not to meant to illustrate that inhalers are bad. In fact, they can save your child's life and it is important that you be willing to use them when necessary. But keep in mind that you must not stop the treatment once the symptoms are removed. When your child has stopped wheezing, begin proactive measures on a regular basis, even when your child is healthy. If your child gets sick and needs an inhaler, use it—but don't stop there. Shortly thereafter it is critical to use herbs that will naturally open the airways, remove the excessive mucus, and heal the irritated mucous membranes.

Doctors are not to blame for the rise in asthma rates and the inability to treat its cause. They are trained to remove symptoms. Parents need the knowledge and confidence to treat imbalances like asthma long before they arise. Even if a condition is genetic, according to Ayurveda, in many cases it can be prevented or cured with home care and vigilance.

Possible Treatments for a Spring Kid-Type Asthmatic Child

Turmeric
There are a few extremely important herbal remedies every parent should know when dealing with irritated mucous membranes. Turmeric is one of these. To date, it's recognized in the scientific lit-

erature to be the most powerful non-steroidal anti-inflammatory herb. Not only is it a classic cold remedy in herbal traditions around the world, but in Ayurvedic medicine it is rarely left out of a cold or upper-respiratory formulation. Turmeric is the very bright orange spice that is most commonly used in Indian or Asian cuisine. It is also the spice that gives yellow mustard its characteristic color.

Most Americans have no idea what a powerful medicine lies right under their noses in the their household spice cabinet. Turmeric is a natural anti-inflammatory with vulnerary, or tissue repair, properties. Not only does it remove excess mucus and reduce inflammation in the sinuses and respiratory tract, it also helps heal and repair damaged and irritated cells. Interestingly, turmeric is also indicated for inflammatory bowel syndromes like Crohn's disease, irritable bowel syndrome, and ulcerative colitis. This is extremely significant for two reasons. First, most anti-inflammatory drugs aggravate the digestive tract in existing inflammatory bowel diseases while turmeric not only reduces inflammation but also heals and repairs cells. Second, the sinuses and the intestinal tract have very similar types of mucous membranes. So turmeric, while repairing cellular intestinal damage, will also heal and restore normal function to the mucosa in the respiratory tract. This important relationship between intestinal and respiratory health is one I will cover in Chapter 4.

Turmeric is also considered to be one of the more powerful natural antibiotics; but unlike most prescribed antibiotics that destroy the good bacteria and flora in the intestines, turmeric actually promotes the growth of good bacteria.

How To Take Turmeric

The best way for your child to take turmeric is to mix equal parts of the powdered herb with raw honey into a paste. Make enough of the paste in advance to last for a day or two. (This paste does not need to be refrigerated.)

Note: Do not feed honey to children before the age of two. Honey can often be contaminated with small amounts of botulin toxin, which is easily broken down in a mature digestive system, but can cause food poisoning or botulism in infants.

At the very first sign of a cold, give your child 1 teaspoon every hour for the first few hours until symptoms subside. After that, take it three to six times a day until the cold is resolved. This usually stops a cold in its tracks. For a severe and chronic cold or respiratory infection, take 1 teaspoon of the paste every two waking hours for up to seven days. In most cases, it will need to be taken frequently for only one to two days.

If, after the first day of taking turmeric, your child is showing no signs of improvement—take him or her to your doctor.

Kid's Dosage: This is a general dosage formula that works for almost all herbal recommendations.

Age in years/20=portion of adult dose

For example, to calculate an 8-year-old child's dose:

8/20 = 8/20ths or 2/5ths (40%) of the adult dose.

Sitopladi

Sitopladi is an important Ayurvedic herbal preparation used to support lung function and reduce and liquefy mucus in the lungs and sinuses. Unlike many of the herbal or allopathic medications used to alleviate a runny nose or reduce congestion (which achieve dry out the mucous membranes), sitopladi reduces congestion by healing, lubricating, and repairing the mucous membranes. The herbs in this classic formulation are: bamboo manna (*Bambusa arundinacia*), long pepper (*Piper longum*), cardamom, cinnamon, and rock sugar. These ingredients combine the demulcent or lubricating properties of rock sugar and cardamom with the mucus liquefying properties of long pepper and cinnamon. Sitopladi reduces excess mucus and congestion without drying out the sinuses, which are susceptible to re-infection—meaning another trip to the doctor.

Sitopladi is particularly effective for asthma and lower-lung and bronchial infections.

How To Take Sitopladi

Sitopladi is typically available as a powdered herbal formula. Mix 1 teaspoon of sitopladi with raw honey into a paste and take 1/2 to 1 teaspoon of the paste three to six times a day between (not with) meals. This paste can be taken as often as needed, even while your child is using an inhaler. Take 1 teaspoon every hour until the difficulties subside. Fortunately, sitopladi actually tastes quite good (due to the rock sugar and the sweet taste of cardamom and cinnamon) and most children have no difficulty with or resistance to taking this frequently to treat a cold or breathing difficulty.

For a Cold in Both the Lungs and Sinuses

When the cold is the sinuses and the congestion moves into the chest, the combination of sitopladi with turmeric and raw honey has an even more powerful effect. Often a cold starts in the sinuses and builds up in the lungs and bronchioles via post-nasal drip. A child with this kind of cold likely experiences a cough and a runny nose. The combination of sitopladi and turmeric treats the mucous membranes and inflammation in the lungs and the sinuses.

How To Take Sitopladi and Turmeric

The herbs can be taken either separately or together by making a paste with raw honey. This combined formula can be taken in the same dosage and frequency as sitopladi alone: 1 teaspoon of the paste every one or two hours as needed for asthma, sinus infection, cold, cough, or flu.

If you are concerned about the amount of honey your child is consuming as a result of frequent doses of the herb/honey paste for a cold, the two herbs can be taken by mixing them with hot or warm water or maple syrup.

Trikatu

For upper-respiratory and sinus infections, trikatu is required knowledge for parents. It's a combination of three herbs: black pepper, long pepper, and ginger. It, too, is best mixed with honey into a paste. It's a bit spicy, so use more honey and use only 1/4 teaspoon of the herb every hour for four to six hours at the first onset of a sore throat, runny nose, or sinus infection. Because of its spiciness, it's very effective for mucus production. Trikatu can be combined with sitopladi to be given when your child has an upper-respiratory infection with a lower respiratory cough. In Chapter 4, trikatu's benefits for healthy digestion are described in detail.

Herbal Review:

Trikatu–Upper-sinus infections and sore throats

Sitopladi–Lower-respiratory infections with cough or asthma

Turmeric–Helps the body eliminate infections and excess mucus in the upper and lower respiratory system

---

Pass the Honey, Honey!

Honey is not only a sweetener used to make herbal mixtures taste good; it is a powerful Ayurvedic medicine. One of its actions is emulsifying mucus, but it also helps to carry other nutrients and herbal medicines into the deeper tissues.

If your children have a fever along with any of the respiratory conditions mentioned—or if they do not show significant improvement in one to two days of using these herbs, take them to your doctor.

Honey should always be eaten raw and never cooked. Cooked honey causes mucus to harden, making it difficult to remove from the body; raw honey breaks up, liquefies, and removes excess mucus.

Raw Honey: There is a considerable difference between raw and cooked honey. Dr. Michael Schmidt tells the following story of a compelling example of the importance of raw honey in his book *Healing Childhood Ear Infections.* Beekeepers typically spray a solution of raw honey and water on beehives to calm the bees. A study was done comparing the use of raw versus pasteurized or cooked honey on beehives. When a solution of pasteurized honey was used, all of the bees exposed died within 20 minutes! Most grocery or health food stores carry raw or uncooked honey. Be sure to read the label carefully to determine if it is raw or cooked.

The Voice of Experience

One of the comforting things about using a 5,000-year-old system of medicine is that there has been time to work out the bugs. Ayurveda is based on careful observation, and over time people have noted the effects of herbs and foods. Somewhere along the line they realized that cooked honey was harmful, so they used only raw honey in their food and medicines. Today, we watch medicines come on and off the market in just a few short years. Imagine how much we would know and how well our medicines would work if they were designed based on 5,000 years of experience!

Winter Woes

Winter kid-types are the next most susceptible to developing colds and other respiratory conditions. Just as winter weather is generally dry and cold, Winter kid-types have a greater tendency to be dry and cold. Nature has its ways of combating the severe cold and dryness of winter. For instance, squirrels eat nuts in the winter not only because they are available, but also because they are oily, demulcent, and lubricating. As discussed already, foods with a higher fat content have a greater insulating and lubricating effect. These high-fat foods are naturally eaten in the winter, both by squirrels and by humans, to keep from becoming excessively dried out.

The extent of the dryness we experience in the winter determines

> The more your child feels dried out in the winter, the more likely it is that the mucous membranes in the respiratory tract will become irritated and make reactive mucus.

the degree to which our body generates excessive reactive mucus in both winter and spring.

So the child who is more susceptible to the woes of cold and flu season in December and January, and dry sinuses in February, is therefore more likely to succumb to the pollen allergies and breathing difficulties—due to excessive mucus—that are so common in the spring.

Health Is Only Skin Deep

Winter kid-types run the risk—especially during the winter months—of becoming excessively dry. Dryness is something much more serious than just the easily visible dry, cracked skin. When the skin becomes dry, the sinuses are also dry, and the cervical lymphatic vessels that drain the sinuses become stagnant. Since the majority of the immune system's vital white blood cells circulate through the lymphatic system, our immunity becomes compromised when lymphatic vessels dry out and lymphatic fluid slows down and becomes more viscous. If the lymphatic fluid becomes slow and boggy, then it is as if the entire immune system is stuck in traffic. Even though the immune system may know that there is a potential cold or flu brewing in the sinuses, it can't get there.

If we want to ward off the chronic and debilitating colds, flus, allergies, and breathing difficulties kids so commonly get, then keeping the sinuses lubricated and the lymphatic system moving is critical. When the movement of fluid through the lymphatic system becomes slow, the body can more easily become overly sensitive and hyperactive to pollens, pollutants, and foods.

The lymphatic system is the primary collector and remover of waste from the body tissues and vital organs. Imagine if you did not remove the trash from your house for months. You would become irritated with the dirty, messy, toxic environment and you would have difficulty cooking meals in the kitchen. You would also lose your taste for the foods that were sitting around rotting in the house. You would feel uncomfortable in your home and unable maintain proper nourishment.

When the lymphatic system becomes slow and sluggish, a similar process occurs in the body. Waste products and toxins build up in the tissues and the body becomes hypersensitive to any toxin, irritant, or pollutant. This is a common cause of allergies. In this type of situation, some children may develop asthma, while others catch colds, and the rest contract allergies.

The Ayurvedic word for lymph is *rasa*. Interestingly, in Sanskrit, this is the same word for taste and emotions. Clearly, the lymphatic system's effect on the body is comprehensive. *Rasa,* in an Ayurvedic sense, is a word that describes the body's fluids. In particular, *rasa* is the body fluid which serves as the first building block for the other major structural tissues of the body including: blood, fat, muscle, nerves, bone, and reproductive tissue. A lymphatic imbalance directly affects the quality production of these important tissues in the body.

The first step in keeping the lymphatic system on its trash collection and removal route is not to let the body dry out. One proactive practice parents can teach their children—as well as practice themselves—is the ancient massage technique called *abhyanga*.

Why Massage?

It's easy to notice that your child's skin becomes drier in the winter. But what we don't see is that the deeper layers of the skin and the tissues beneath them can also become dry. Too much dryness causes the skin to lose the ability to function as an organ. When supple, moist, and in balance, the skin drains toxins and waste products efficiently into the lymphatic system; which then carries the waste away from the skin and out of the body. If the skin stops functioning, the lymphatic fluid will also stagnate and the waste will begin to back up in the skin. Along with the liver and kidneys, the skin is one of our primary organs of both processing and eliminating toxins. With the amount of pollution our skin is exposed to and the chemicals people slather on their skin in the form of lotions, creams, cosmetics, and sunscreens, you can imagine how important the skin's drainage into the lymphatic system can be.

When the skin is supple and well-lubricated for extended periods of time, the lymphatic system moves freely, allowing the disease-fighting white blood cells of the immune system also to move freely. But, if dry skin interferes with the removal of waste products, the lymphatic fluid stagnates and the immune system becomes compromised.

Dry skin soon loses its luster and starts to sag, and waste removal and the immune system are compromised. In kids, this usually results in a skin rash, allergic hives, or eczema. One of the most effective ways to treat and prevent all-too-common dry skin is with a simple daily massage for your child. A daily massage can lubricate both superficial and deep layers of the skin, restoring normal circulation, waste removal, and other functions.

Parental Tip: Dry skin in children is a warning sign of other imbalances in the body. Daily massage using moisturizers which lubricate the deep tissues of the skin and restore lymphatic drainage will help bring the rest of the body into balance.

What To Put on the Skin?

Unfortunately, many lotions that make the skin look good on the surface are filled with synthetic and non-absorbing chemicals, many of which are carcinogenic when ingested. Few of us are aware of just how many toxic chemicals are in the personal care products we use. A 1989 United States House of Representatives Report found that 884 chemicals used in personal care products were toxic: 146 cause tumors, 218 cause reproductive complications, 778 cause acute toxicity, 314 cause biological mutations and 376 cause skin irritations. I will discuss the issue of toxic chemicals in the home in more detail in Chapter 8.

Most skin care products are designed to make the skin look better with no consideration for maintaining the healthy function of the skin as an organ. These synthetic foreign substances can obstruct the small lymph-drainage channels in the deeper layers of the skin, inhibiting the skin from functioning optimally as an organ. What makes things confusing is that products are often labeled and marketed in a misleading way; "all natural" doesn't always mean that it is good for you. So how should a responsible parent read labels? Look for products without preservatives and with simple understandable ingredients, rather than chemicals you have never heard of. These are ideal for maintaining optimal skin health.

Ayurveda recommends the use of warm sesame or other oils on the skin. Oils tend to pull impurities out of the deep layers of the skin, acting as detoxifiers and allowing the skin to function effectively as an organ. When the skin is functioning optimally, it will allow the body's natural moisturizing factors to lubricate the skin. Certain kid-types, like winter types, often need to use moisturizers. Oils might not be the best option for keeping the skin well-moisturized. The lipid molecules in most oils are too large to penetrate the thick keratin and softer phospholipid barriers of the skin. I prefer to use natural butters such as shea, mango, avocado, coconut, and other butters. These natural butters have smaller molecules that can penetrate the pores of the skin into the deeper tissues, effectively moisturizing all the layers of the skin.

> When oils are used they should be cold-pressed and can be medicated with specific herbs designed to restore function to and help detoxify or purify the skin.

Abhyanga

Ayurveda recommends massage with warm oil before bathing each day. I am sure parents cannot envision themselves massaging their children every morning before school; however, you can teach your children how to do a self-massage. Self-massage can be done right in the shower. After washing and shampooing, while the shower is still running, your children can take a small amount of sesame or other high-quality, cold-pressed oil or butter and rub it all over their body like a lotion. When the skin is wet, a small amount of oil easily covers the entire body without leaving a heavy greasy feeling. When your children leave the shower they can towel dry and the skin will be moisturized all day as if they used an expensive lotion.

Getting your children into this habit can be a simple yet incredibly powerful tool for helping them maintain optimal health. A few educational showers may be needed to train your children, but it should be easy as children are like monkeys—monkey see, monkey do. If you as a parent develop the habit of self-massage, often your children will model this behavior on their own.

On weekends when you have more time, you can spread towels on the bathroom floor and give yourself and your children or infant a full-body warm-oil massage. I have never met a child who did not like to be touched, and this can be a time to support skin and immune system health while bonding with your child. Studies have shown an increase in production of growth hormones in subjects who were touched regularly compared to those who were not.

Usually kids relax as soon as the warm oil hits their backs. Our kids want it to last all day. However, there will always be times when your kids simply do not want to be still, and their massage will need to be postponed. You can heat the oil by running the bottle of oil under hot water or setting the bottle in a bowl of hot (not boiling) water. Make sure the room is warm, but not too hot; it is best to do the massage in a room warmed by the sun.

> Massage is not just kid-stuff; it is a great technique for keeping adult skin soft, supple, and healthy.

How To Give an Ayurvedic Massage

- Classically you would start with the child sitting up. First massage the head. If you have time you can put the oil right into the child's hair and firmly massage the scalp.
- With the child sitting, work your way down the shoulders, heart, chest and mid-back areas using sweeping strokes.
- Then have the child lie down on his or her stomach. If time

permits you can spend more time massaging the back and shoulders.

- Move on to give a strong hand and finger massage.
- From the hands move up the arm to the shoulder. Use circular strokes around the wrist, elbow, and shoulder joints, and long back-and-forth strokes on the long bones of the upper arm and forearm.
- Then massage the hips with circular strokes working your way down to the feet. Use long back-and-forth strokes on the long bones and circular strokes on the knee and ankle joints.
- Do an extended foot massage with vigorous strokes to both the bottoms and tops of the feet.
- Turn your child over onto the back and massage the feet again. This is where many of the nerves in the body begin and end, so massaging the feet has a calming effect on the entire nervous system. Be sure to massage each toe as well—children love it!
- Work your way up the front of the leg as before.
- Massage with gentle clockwise circular strokes over the abdomen.
- Massage around each side of the chest area.
- Massage the shoulders, arms, and hands again.
- Finish with a sweeping massage stroke up the arms, down the torso, down the legs, and off the feet.
- Cover your child with a towel and let him or her rest.

In traditional cultures this type of massage is given daily to children starting the day they are born.

Summer in the City

Summer kid-types are not big mucus-makers as children. They are the hot, fiery, competitive ones who are not overly fond of the sun or getting overheated. They are usually kicking off the blankets at night while the winter kid-types can't pile enough covers on to stay warm. Summer kid-types typically have a better-than-average immune system. Their circulation is great, their digestion is strong, and they possess the mental drive to push through things like colds, along with any other obstacles that stand in their way. Fortunately, there are few pure summer kid-types, and these qualities, which can be intense, are almost always softened by the more sensitive qualities of winter or the more stable qualities of spring.

Summer kid-types are usually thrown off balance by an accumulation of heat. This heat intolerance doesn't usually become noticeable until their teens, 20s, and 30s when they complain of acne, heart burn, and a variety of other inflammatory conditions. When summer kid-types tend to catch fewer than average colds that are usually not as intense. When summer kid-types get overheated, their skin resembles the desert's surface—dry and parched. Their lips and feet chafe and crack and they can be susceptible to skin rashes. Their mucous membranes can become dry and irritated, beginning the process of making reactive mucus. They are then more susceptible to seasonal colds.

The cold-remedy herbs I mentioned for the winter and spring kid-types—turmeric and sitopladi preparations—are effective for any kid-type, including the hot summer kid-types, when the cold is due to bacteria or viruses breeding in sinuses which are producing excessive mucus.

Heat Wave

Although summer kid-types are not as susceptible to catching colds, they still do, and consequently there are a few rules of prevention. When summer kid-types become unbalanced due to overheating the body or mind from stress, overwork at school, taking life too seriously, an excess of physical activity, too much heat or sun, or eating excessive amounts of spicy or salty foods, heat can accumulate in their body and through the skin for elimination. This rising heat can be an underlying cause of teenage acne and other skin conditions.

Before they reach acne stages, summer kid-types are likely to complain of skin rashes and allergies. Acne is typically caused by a set of imbalances and is treated by cooling the body and supporting proper digestion and elimination. The strong, hot digestion of summer kid-types are susceptible to overheating, making them complain of loose bowel movements. This is an indication that digestion has become too hot and the digestive fire is in fact lique-fying the stool and potentially inflaming the intestinal wall. This heat will inflame the intestinal mucosa, triggering the production of reactive mucus. The buildup of mucus along the intestinal wall obstructs proper assimilation of food, and both the blood and lym-phatic drainage of the intestines can become sluggish and toxic. This toxicity causes lymphatic stagnation leading to the circula-tion of impurities in the bloodstream. The skin then gets used as a primary means of removing this waste, eliciting a variety of chronic skin rashes, including acne.

Earlier I discussed the importance of the interconnected skin and lymphatic system and the need for lubrication and moisture. Since summer kid-types are prone to drying out from excessive heat, their skin and the lymphatic drainage beneath the skin can dry out. If the skin is excessively dry, eczema, a dry irritated skin rash, can form. If the lymphatic fluid is affected and the child has a ten-dency to make mucus or is a summer-spring kid-type, then a skin allergy like hives may be triggered. It is important to heal the skin and clear the stagnation in the lymphatic system through treatment.

When the lymphatic system slows down and the immune system becomes compromised, the body is not only more suscep-tible to colds but it can become hypersensitive to pollutants, pol-lens, and other respiratory irritants. There may be digestive issues and other factors that will contribute to your child's allergies and skin rashes. Remember, getting the lymphatic system moving is a principal requirement for optimal health.

Manjistha

Manjistha is an herb that is beneficial for both the skin and the lym-phatic system. It is known to break up stagnation in the lymphatic system, purify the blood and provide support for a variety of skin conditions. Manjistha (*Rubia cordifolia*) can be found in capsules or as a powder. It is an extremely safe herb that helps revive restoring lymphatic circulation and function, an effective immune system, improved skin quality, and an overall sense of well-being.

How To Take Manjistha

The normal dose of manjistha for a child is 300–500 milligrams two times a day with water, after meals, or on an empty stomach.

Jason

Jason was a 5-year-old boy who came to me with a chronic mumps-like swelling in a lymph gland in his neck. He had suffered with this condition going on three months when his parents brought him in. He had been to numerous doctors, none of whom succeeded in removing the lump. I suggested that Jason take manjistha to improve his lymphatic circulation and reduce the swelling. Within three days his parents reported that the lump had significantly improved, and by the week's end the swollen lymph gland was back to normal.

Manjistha is a powerful herb that is safe for both children and adults. It is not a cold-fighter or antibiotic, but it can be important in fighting both colds and infections as it restores the body's lymphatic function, allowing the body to fight the infection on its own. The lymphatic system is one of the most important and least understood systems of the human body. As a result, most lymphatic-based conditions go unnoticed and often untreated.

> Lymphatic imbalances are often chronic. They have taken time to develop and they will take time to clear up; a child may need to take manjistha for one to three months before the imbalance is fully resolved.

Chapter 4

Secret 3—Colds Start in the Digestive System

I t is a common misconception that kids have iron-clad digestive systems. On the contrary, children complain of tummyaches more often than colds and earaches; their digestive systems are particularly susceptible to upset as their little stomachs and intestines take a while to get the hang of things. Although tummyaches are common, they are not well-publicized because they are usually short-lived in children, and don't typically result in doctor's visits and antibiotics. At worst, children moan for a while, throw up, or experience diarrhea, and before you know it they're back in action. But digestive problems can cause disorders in the body that are not as apparent but much more insidious.

In this chapter, I will describe some of the more common causes of stomachaches, constipation, and other digestive imbalances. Ailments of the digestive system cause 80% of all childhood diseases. This chapter will help you notice and evaluate warning signs, apply preventive techniques, and treat, when indicated, the most common childhood digestive imbalances. We will discuss how symptoms vary among kid-types. We will look beyond the symptoms to understand the mechanisms that underly these imbalances and how they also contribute to the root cause of many other

Knowing how to look for the root cause of a problem is the key to getting off the roller coaster of treatments which merely remove the symptoms today before they return with a vengeance tomorrow.

problems in the body, such as skin rashes, allergies, and colds.

Understanding these mechanisms is powerful information for parents. For instance, if you can recognize that the underlying cause of a skin rash is an imbalance in the digestive system, therapies can be directed toward eliminating the cause rather than suppressing the symptoms.

The Intestinal Everglades

Remember that young children are in the spring, Kapha, or mucus-making time of their lives. This is significant not only in the respiratory system; the linings of both the digestive system and the sinuses have similar mucous membranes. When the sinuses produce excessive mucus, the stomach and intestines commonly do the same. This mucus tends to create a bogginess in the stomach and intestines which slows the digestive process. Children are especially susceptible to this bogginess, both due to their tendency to make excess mucus and because their ability to produce digestive acids and enzymes has not yet fully developed.

An appropriate amount of mucus is crucial to the healthy functioning of the digestive system. Just the right amount of intestinal mucus allows the food bolus or meal to move easily through the small and large intestines. Too much mucus compromises the assimilation of food and essential nutrients, while not enough can render the intestinal wall hypersensitive to irritants like spicy foods, preservatives, food dyes, hard-to-digest foods, and the stomach's own acids.

Just as the cause of many respiratory conditions is the excessive production of mucus, the cause of many digestive complaints is excessive production and accumulation of mucus. Monitoring digestive mucus is an essential aspect of parents' efforts to maintain the strength of their children's digestion. Both monitoring mucus and maintaining appropriate levels of mucus are difficult tasks because the standard American diet is filled with mucus-producing foods.

Say "Aahh," Please!

How do you go about monitoring digestive mucus and the health and strength of the digestive tract? Say "Aahh!" Modern doctors ask their patients to stick out their tongues to glean information about the possibility of an infection, but practitioners in traditional medical systems have used tongue diagnosis for thousands of years to assess the internal status of the body. The tongue is the beginning of our very long digestive system. Ayurveda teaches that the state of affairs of the entire digestive system can be examined by a quick and simple look at the tongue, just like checking under the hood of a car. The condition of the tongue can give parents some basic information about their child's well-being.

Most people think that a normal tongue is bright red and clear with no coating whatsoever. In fact, a normal tongue is pinkish in color with a slight whitish film. Its texture is soft and fairly uniform. But how often do we see healthy pink tongues? All too often, the tongue is covered with a thick mucusy coating; or is flaming bright red. The condition of the tongue is one of our strongest tools to tell us about problems quietly brewing below the surface.

Weeks before a cold or asthma attack manifests, a digestive problem might be developing in the large intestine. If this is the case, the coating on the tongue changes in color from a healthy pink to an unhealthy white. When kids get sick, we observe this heavy, toxic coating...along with the hard-to-miss horrendous breath.

If a tongue is wet, slimy, mucusy, or covered with a thick coating, then these are good indications that the entire digestive system is congested due to excessive production of mucus. In Ayurvedic terms, this heavy white coating, called *ama*, is a sign of accumulated undigested food and toxic material. Excess *ama* on the tongue is one of the first signs of toxicity and a cold-in-the-making. We can counteract this condition by strengthening and supporting the upper digestion and by removing the accumulated mucus from the lining of the small and large intestines. I will discuss treatment for this type of imbalance in the section on spring digestion.

A tongue that is dry or cracked, especially in a child who is constantly thirsty, can indicate dehydration, dryness of the mucous membranes of the intestinal lining, and constipation. I will address this common imbalance in the discussion of winter digestion. On the other hand, a tongue that is bright red, scarlet, or even purplish in color indicates the presence of too much heat or acidity in the digestive system. The mucous membranes are likely to be inflamed and irritated; and the stool is often chronically loose. I will address this imbalance when I discuss summer digestion.

The Tongue as a Map

As people have observed the tongue over millennia, certain sections of the tongue have consistently reflected problems in corresponding areas of the digestive system. The map of the tongue shows the lower part of the digestive system, the large intestine, toward the back of the tongue. A thick and heavy coating in this area reveals an imbalance or a buildup of *ama* in the large intestine. On the center line and about midway to the back of the tongue, the upper portion of the digestive system, the stomach, is typically reflected. An increased coating in middle of the tongue indicates a buildup of mucus and congestion in the stomach. Between the stomach and the large intestine areas is the region that represents the small intestine. It is in the small intestine that most of the assimilation of nutrients takes place, so coating in this area indicates a problem with the body's ability to efficiently absorb nutrition from food.

Another important clue to read on the tongue's map is the presence of scallops, which look like teeth marks along the sides or edge of the tongue. These can indicate malabsorption. A quick glance at your child's tongue on a regular basis can be an invaluable tool for monitoring his or her digestion in real time and making a proactive plan for perfect health for your kids.

The Tongue Is a Mirror of the Gastrointestinal Tract.

Diagram of one's own tongue (as seen in a mirror)

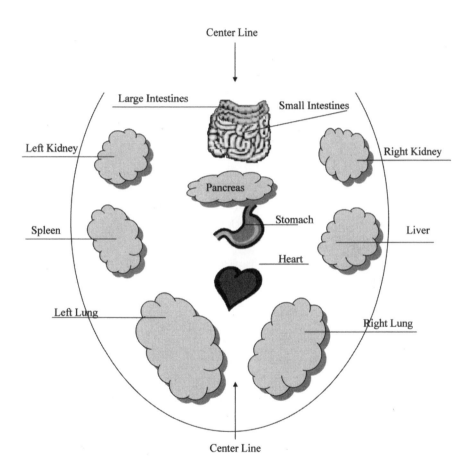

TONGUE MAP

Have You Scraped Your Tongue Lately? Teach your children the art of tongue scraping. You may think: why would anyone want to scrape their tongue and what would you use? Cleaning the tongue is a well-known technique used throughout the world. In many parts of Europe and Asia children are taught at a young age to scrape their tongue first thing in the morning as a part of their morning hygiene. This is as essential as brushing their teeth or washing their hair.

Just as the skin all over the body is a major organ for detoxification, the tongue is a major vehicle for detoxification of the digestive system. When toxins start building up in the digestive system, the body uses the tongue as a means of removing them—the result is a coated tongue. This is why the tongue develops a coating when a child is sick. By cleaning or scraping the tongue you can remove these toxins and help the body process more toxins if necessary.

Scraping the tongue is also important because it is unwise to allow a collection of toxins to sit in the mouth all day breeding millions of bacteria. Scraping the tongue can be used to help cure a child's bad breath and support healthier dental hygiene.

You can buy a tongue scraper inexpensively in most health food stores or use the upside-down edge of a soup spoon.

Stress and the Stomach

We usually think of stress as an adult malady, with childhood being a time of idyllic stress-free days. But, unfortunately, children are subject to stress—and are extremely susceptible to it. Wondering who they are going to sit next to during recess can be more stressful for children than significant adult stressors. A child's stomach is often the target for this stress. It is important for parents to recognize how their children handle the stress of going to school, interacting with other children, and keeping up with their studies. The digestive system—particularly the stomach—can be one of the first places in the body where the effects of stress show themselves.

Winter, or Vata, kid-types are typically sensitive, and they tend to let everyone know how well they are handling—or not handling—

stress. They may not always tell you in words, but their actions are conclusive. Their delicate nervous systems feel almost everything, unlike the other kid-types who possess thicker skins. Winter kid-types run a greater risk of the stress they feel impacting their digestive systems, making them more susceptible to tummyaches and digestive complaints.

Summer kid-types may express the impact of stress by becoming angry or irritable. A parent may find them acting out this stress against a sibling or a close friend. Because their digestive systems are typically more robust than other types, it may take more time—or more stress—for childhood pressures to impact their digestion. And when it does, they may feel the effects of heat, inflammation, and acidity in the form of heartburn, loose stools, malabsorption, and indigestion.

Spring kid-types tend to internalize their stress and not talk about it much. Parents have to carefully watch spring kid-types. You might only notice chronic breathing difficulty, moodiness, fatigue, or complacency. The stress will affect their digestion without the initial presence of noticeable symptoms, but beneath the surface they will build up increasing bogginess or heaviness. This can slow down the digestive process causing malabsorption and problems with circulation, both in the lymphatic system and in the bloodstream. They may hold onto more water and gain weight or eat more when they become stressed out.

Secret 3: The third health secret is early detection of digestive problems and the knowledge of how to bring your child's digestion back into balance with proper herbs and diet. It is a powerful preventive technique in the quest for perfect health for your kids. By evaluating their digestive systems, you can monitor their current and future health. Ayurvedic medicine attributes 80% of all disease to a malfunctioning digestive system. Instead of waiting for a cold or other illness to arrive, noticing the early warning signs of the digestive system will be a tip-off for parents that a cold is in the making.

Spring Kid-Type Digestion

Just as we saw in the respiratory system, certain body types will make more digestive mucus then other types. Unsurprisingly, spring kid-types run the risk of having a heavier and slower digestive system with a greater tendency for excessive mucus production when compared to the other types. Spring kid-types should take extra precautions to limit foods that create mucus.

As we have mentioned, some foods that are prone to encouraging mucus production are:

- dairy products
- fast foods
- fried foods
- ice-cold foods
- cold drinks
- pasta and bread

In the damp spring months, spring kid-types, who are already in their spring lifecycle (childhood) and who make a habit of eating Mac 'n' Cheese or pizza for dinner with cold milk, followed by milkshakes or ice cream for dessert, will no doubt produce excess mucus in their digestive systems. This mucus can stick to the intestinal wall, creating a dirty-filter effect of clogging up the membranes that allow the passage of nutrients into the bloodstream and the lymphatic fluid, thereby slowing the digestive process and compromising proper absorption and assimilation of nutrients.

We move food and remove waste products through the intestinal tract with a series of muscular contractions called peristalsis. Excessive mucus coating the lining of the intestinal wall can compromise peristalsis because the mucus is too heavy for the smooth muscle of the intestines to contract against. This results in slow and boggy digestive and eliminative processes. For this reason, it is important to know the type and appropriate dietary considerations of your child. In Chapter 7, I will review family-friendly grocery lists that whet the appetite of any hungry kid-type.

Because of the naturally slow metabolism of spring kid-types, their digestion can also be slow so their tendency to produce excess mucus can create digestive problems. How many times have parents heard the words, "Mommy, I have a tummyache." Sometimes these tummyaches are caused by a temporary standstill in the digestive system, which can occur when a child is overly stressed out or has overeaten a heavy, mucus-producing meal. This standstill can cause mucus to build up in the slow and boggy intestines, leading to headaches, stomachaches, and nausea. At this point, the best thing can often be to let the child vomit rather than suppress the symptoms with anti-nausea medications. Throwing up is often the body's way of expelling excess mucus and curing a tummyache.

One of my daughters, now 13, has never caught a cold. When she becomes ill, she gets a headache, then a stomachache, and finally throws up. In less than three to five hours, or after a night's sleep, she is back to normal, feeling better and clearer than she was before getting sick. Her body and digestive system are very sensitive, and she vomits as a method of detoxification, responding to bad foods or excessive stress. Her sensitive system does not allow the buildup of impurities in the large intestine which would be absorbed into the lymphatic fluid, thus compromising her immune system. By vomiting when necessary, she gets rid of this waste immediately. The only down side to her body's cleansing process is that she frequently gets detox headaches and tummyaches.

Throwing up is not always a bad thing for the body to do—it is a natural response when the body needs to get rid of toxins, contaminated food, or excessive mucus. This can often be a child's best medicine.

Note: It is important to notice how often your child is throwing up. Frequent vomiting can be indicative of more serious medical problems, requiring the advice of a physician. Recurrent vomiting can also be a sign of eating disorders, which are unfortunately appearing more frequently in younger and younger children.

Tummyache and Colic Formula

You can use this formula to help the stomach settle down and recover when your child has a tummyache, stomach problems, or colic.

Use:

- 1/2 teaspoon of fennel powder
- 1/2 teaspoon of cumin powder
- 1/10th teaspoon or small pinch of hing, or asafoetida (a substitute for onion that helps to decrease gas and bloating)

How To Take Colic Formula

1. Combine the three herbs to make a powder.
2. Boil 2 cups of water combined with the powdered herbs down to 1 cup.
3. Filter through a cheesecloth and save the liquid.
4. Give 10 to 20 drops of the liquid every five to ten minutes until the tummyache subsides.

Herbal Support for Spring Digestion

To help spring kid-types digest their food and eliminate wastes more effectively, there are a number of herbs that help the stomach break down hard-to-digest and mucus-producing foods. These herbs, recipes, and formulations are very effective in supporting a more robust upper-digestive system. I will provide several recipes and formulas that all have a similar effect. It is valuable to have multiple options for strengthening digestion as kids can be a little finicky when it comes to ingesting medicines.

Trikatu to the Rescue

The first digestive herbal formula I will discuss is called *trikatu,* which works well for kids with a heavy white coating on the tongue.

Occasionally, in our house, we will rent a movie, order pizza, and enjoy this very hard-to-digest meal at eight o'clock at night. (Eating later in the evening is hard on the digestion; after the sun sets the digestive system, along with the metabolism, slows down in order to prepare the body for sleep.) This combination of foods, especially in the evening, is one of the quickest ways to create an environment of both intestinal and respiratory mucus production that could breed a child's next cold. To counteract this, our children are not allowed to eat their pizza or start the movie until they have taken trikatu. Trikatu helps counteract the mucus-producing and digestive-slowing effects of dairy, eating late at night, or eating cold food. It is also one of the cold-fighting herbs mentioned in chapter 3.

- Trikatu is a combination of three digestive herbs: ginger, black pepper, and long pepper.
- This classic Ayurvedic formulation was developed some 3,000 to 4,000 years ago and is now commonly available in most health food stores.
- Each of these herbs individually helps to increase the production of stomach acids and enzymes while liquefying any excess mucus. When these herbs are combined, their effectiveness is greatly enhanced.

How To Take Trikatu

Children may take one or two capsules depending on their age (a good rule of thumb is one capsule for younger children and two for older children) with a heavy, hard-to-digest meal to ward off indigestion and excess mucus production. Trikatu is spicy and heating, so you want to give two capsules only if the meal is especially hard to digest, large, late in the evening, or eaten by a spring kid-type with strong digestion who is famous for producing excess mucus.

Trikatu can also be used by mixing equal parts of powered herb and honey into a paste and taking 1/2 teaspoon of the paste before meals.

This formula is particularly effective for spring kid-types who tend to have heavy and slow digestion. These kids can take this formula before all meals (not just pizza) if needed during times of excess mucus production. For a spring kid-type this may be indicated throughout the spring season and possibly in the cold and flu season of January and February.

Trikatu can be used safely by all kid-types with all meals. If a child has loose stools after using trikatu, reduce the amount of herb or number of capsules given. This rarely happens, but when it does, it is due to the spicy nature of trikatu.

For those late-night pizzas eaten when very few digestive systems have the strength necessary to completely break down all that cheese, trikatu is a perfect choice for the entire family.

Caution: This is not an endorsement for eating pizza or ice cream daily, or regularly scheduling the evening meal at eight o'clock accompanied by trikatu. This is only suggested as a remedy for those rare late night pizza (or other mucusy food) deliveries.

More Natural Digestive Boosters

Ginger Pickle

Ginger pickle is a simple and effective means for stimulating upper-digestive fire. It can be used before any meal to help strengthen digestion and is particularly useful when eating heavy and hard-to-digest foods, or when eating late at night.

To make ginger pickle:

1. Start with a 2-inch piece of fresh ginger root.
2. Peel and slice it into dime-sized pieces.
3. Lay the pieces flat on a plate like little pizzas and sprinkle them with lemon juice and salt.

How To Take Ginger Pickle

Eat one or two slices of the prepared ginger before each meal to boost digestion.

The plate of ginger slices can be sealed with plastic and stored in the refrigerator for up to two weeks. You can also put a few slices in a baggie or container and take them to work with you or send them to school with your kids.

Ginger Honey

The ginger honey recipe takes a little longer to make, but is sweeter and more popular with children. It can be used as an alternative to the trikatu or the ginger pickle.

To make ginger honey:

1. Put a large, clean, unpeeled piece of fresh ginger root through a juicer. (If you don't have a juicer, you can squeeze the ginger in a garlic press and express the juice.)
2. Add a pinch of salt to the juice and mix well.
3. Measure the amount of juice extracted and then add twice as much raw honey as ginger juice.
4. Stir the mixture very well and store in the refrigerator.

How To Take Ginger Honey

Take 1 teaspoon of this liquid before meals to stimulate the digestive fire.

This mixture will stay fresh in the refrigerator in a sealed container for up to one week.

Cooking Spices to Aid Digestion

The spices listed below can be used by incorporating them into foods while cooking. For best results heat the spices in a pan with ghee or olive oil before adding them to a recipe.

You can also make a stock using these digestive herbs and add them to a stir-fry or add to a cooking pot.

To make a stock:

1. Add 1/2 teaspoon of each herb used to 2 cups of water.
2. Boil the mixture until it reduces down to 1 cup liquid.
3. Strain through a fine strainer or cheesecloth.
4. Use this liquid stock to taste in any desired recipe.

The following digestive herbs can be used individually or together and are available in grocery, health food, or Asian grocery stores:

- black mustard seed
- coriander seed
- cumin
- fennel
- ginger
- hing, or asafoetida

Herbs for Other Spring Digestion Maladies

Fenugreek

For spring kid-types who have slow lower digestion, signified by constipation with indigestion and bloating, fenugreek can be very helpful.

- Fenugreek seed (Trigonella foenum) is a warming, bitter herb that is a natural digestive tonic.
- Fenugreek has a unique effect on the body; not only does it liquefy and remove excessive mucus with its pungent taste, but it also heals irritated mucous membranes through its action as a healing and lubricating demulcent herb.
- Cooked with milk, this herb is a classic remedy for children's tummyaches and can also be used to pull mucus off the intestinal wall. Once the mucus is removed, the assimilation of food and the peristalsis (contractibility) of the intestines is greatly enhanced.

To make fenugreek milk:

1. Add 1 teaspoon (1 tablespoon for adults) of fenugreek seed powder to 1 cup of milk.
2. Place in a pot on the stove and bring to a boil.
3. Once the milk is boiling, immediately remove from the heat, let cool, and then drink slowly.
4. This is very soothing and healing for the upper digestion.

Turmeric

Turmeric, known for its antibiotic qualities and respiratory system-supporting properties, also supports digestive strength and is a significant anti-inflammatory herb for the intestinal tract.

Turmeric functions much like fenugreek to both increase digestive strength and to heal and repair the intestinal mucosa. It is particularly useful to reduce excess spring qualities and phlegm in the body. For spring kid-types, turmeric addresses both the inflammation and irritation of the intestinal and respiratory mucosa.

As a cold-fighter this herb is second to none. Although many people think its cold-fighting properties come from its antibacterial and anti-inflammatory nature, in fact turmeric is one of the most effective cold-fighting herbs because of its vulnerary (tissue repairing) properties for the mucous membranes of the intestinal wall. Turmeric helps to improve the intestinal flora and improve all aspects of the digestive process.

How To Take Turmeric

Turmeric mixed with equal amounts of raw honey into a paste is extremely palatable for children.

Children can take 1 teaspoon of this mixture for indigestion or gas. If they are experiencing a cold and indigestion together, turmeric will treat both conditions.

Turmeric can be taken as a milk decoction using the same recipe as described for fenugreek. One teaspoon of turmeric brought to a boil in 1 cup of milk is a soothing remedy for children's digestive complaints.

Why Not Enzymes?

When a child or adult has digestive problems, supplemental digestive enzymes are often recommended. But these enzymes are naturally manufactured in our saliva, stomach, and throughout the digestive system; they are also naturally available in the foods that we eat. Unfortunately, the food available in our grocery stores is less then adequate when it comes to nutritional content. According to the U.S. Department of Agriculture nutrient database, the amount of iron in 100 grams of spinach today is about 1.3 milligrams, compared to 158 milligrams per 100 grams in 1948. That means it would take 120 bowls of spinach today to get the same amount of iron as one bowl in 1948. The year is significant because it was the years following 1948 that chemical fertilizers were introduced to increase yields. Farmers subsequently stopped rotating crops and applying organic fertilizers to the soil. Soon thereafter, the soil began losing many of the trace elements and nutrients essential for optimum health. So it may be true to some extent that our foods today have fewer available enzymes. With this in mind, many doctors are recommending enzymes to their patients for digestive imbalances.

The problem with taking supplemental enzymes is that our bodies naturally make the enzymes that are essential for proper digestion. Taking supplemental digestive enzymes gives the body the message that it does not need to make its own. The more we take enzymes, the fewer enzymes will be produced by the body, and the sooner the digestive system will lose the capacity to manufacture the enzymes on its own. This creates a situation where the body runs the risk of becoming dependent on supplemental enzymes—especially if digestive enzymes are misused.

> I once worked with a patient who was using supplemental digestive enzymes. When he first started, he took two capsules with each meal, but he had to increase the amount continually as his body became more dependent on the supplemental enzymes and less able to produce its own. By the time he came to see me, he needed to take 17 capsules of digestive enzymes with each meal in order to digest his food!

Just as there are times when it is necessary to take antibiotics or other pharmaceuticals to fight an infection or allow the airways to clear, there are times when a course of digestive enzymes may be just the thing to create more strength in the digestive system, for example, during periods of stress. It is important to use them carefully.

The science of Ayurveda gives us many not-so-secret methods to support and improve the body's own ability to take care of itself. The goal of this system is not to create a dependency on herbs or supplements for any condition. Rather, Ayurveda aims to use herbs or other substances to strengthen the body. One example of is the use of herbs that enhance the body's ability to break down hard-to-digest foods by helping it make stronger digestive acids and enzymes. Once the body has reset its digestive ability, it can be gracefully weaned from herbs, leaving the individual free of any dependencies—which is particularly important for our children.

Winter Kid-Type Digestion

Winter kid-types tend to be more restless and delicate compared to the spring and summer kid-types. They are typically light sleepers and are prone to dryness throughout their bodies. Dryness in their skin can develop into eczema, or other dry-skin disorders, if it becomes extreme. Dry skin on the body's surface usually indicates that conditions are right for dryness elsewhere in the body, like the lining of the intestines. This can lead to constipation, and winter kid-types commonly suffer from chronic constipation. As we have discussed previously, dryness, especially if both the sinuses and the intestines become dried out, can lead to relentless production of reactive mucus.

First, it can compromise assimilation and slow the process of elimination as we saw in the unbalanced spring kid-types. But in winter kid-types, we don't see bogginess and heaviness; instead the mucus has a tendency to dry out and harden along the intestinal wall. This hardness not only affects absorption and elimination but makes it very difficult for the intestines to contract effectively, and soon the seeds of chronic constipation are sown.

Why Not Laxatives?

When any of us are constipated, our first thought (once we realize we are constipated, which can sometimes take a while) is to reach for a laxative. But the worst thing you can do for your children's constipation is to give them laxatives. Laxatives work by irritating the bowel, making something as gentle as senna leaf act as an irritant. Laxatives like senna produce their effect in the body by forcing the muscles of the intestines to contract intensely as a result of being irritated by the bitterness. The problem with such laxatives is that the intestinal mucosa soon becomes desensitized and resistant to the irritants. The senna leaf tea that once worked wonders now hardly works at all. Larger, more frequent doses and stronger laxatives are soon necessary for elimination as the constipation becomes chronic.

What's even worse is that the intestinal wall can become desensitized to the normal process of food moving through. Normally, the pressure of the food bolus on the intestinal wall triggers the peristaltic contractions. The overuse of laxatives can lead to the intestinal wall becoming desensitized even to the food bolus, shutting down the regular cycle of digestion and elimination.

The most effective first step in treating constipation is to strengthen the contractibility of the intestinal wall with a bowel *tonic* rather than a bowel-irritating laxative. One such tonic used frequently in Ayurveda is *trifala,* an extremely safe herbal formula.

Trifala

- Trifala is a compound of three dried and powdered fruits—haritaki, bibhitaki, and amalaki—with combined actions to balance the digestive system.
- Botanical Names:
- Haritaki: *Terminalia chebula*
- Bibhitaki: *Terminalia bellierica*
- Amalaki: *Embilica officinalis*

How Trifala Works

Trifala is a bowel tonic that helps the muscular wall of the intestines contract with more effectiveness and vigor. It does not do this through an irritating effect; rather, it both cleanses and tonifies the mucous membranes of the intestinal lining, increasing the motility of the colon. By removing excess mucus buildup, trifala allows the intestines to resume their normal contractibility. Because trifala helps to restore normal functioning, the colon does not develop a dependency to it. If needed, trifala can be used safely for extended periods of time. Even though it is classically used for constipation, it can also be used for diarrhea, thanks to its balancing effect on the digestive system.

The interplay of the three herbs is important as each one balances an excess of one of the seasonal types while at the same time increasing the others. Haritaki is good for all types but primarily balances winter. Bibhitaki balances spring and summer but can increase winter. Amalaki balances summer and winter but increases spring.

Together this combination is good for all three types:

- Haritaki (*Terminalia chebula*): Its name means "Life Giver." Primarily balancing for winter types, its uses include treatment for chronic constipation, nervous disorders, digestion, and it is an effective expectorant.
- Bibhitaki (*Terminalia bellierica*): Most widely used as a tonic for spring types, it has specific actions on the respiratory system. It also acts to remove the excess mucus from the digestive tract allowing for better motility and absorption.
- Amalaki (*Embilica officinalis*): Primarily balancing for summer types, it is effective in dyspepsia, both ulcer and non-ulcer related. Partly because of its high (higher than oranges) Vitamin C content it is a powerful detoxifier and anti-oxidant. It also relieves inflamed tissue in the stomach and intestines.

How To Take Trifala
Taking trifala after meals helps to move the digestive process along without stagnation.

An appropriate dose of trifala is between one and three 500 milligram tablets taken after meals. The amount will depend on the sensitivity of your children and chronicity of their constipation.

For children who cannot swallow tablets, you can use two alternative methods: one is to mix equal parts trifala powder with honey into a paste and take 1 teaspoon after meals; the other is to make a room-temperature decoction or type of tea with the trifala and water. The trifala water can be taken once or twice a day, in the morning and evening, as needed for your child's constipation.

To make trifala water:

1. Add 1 teaspoon of trifala to a glass of water, stir, and let sit overnight.
2. In the morning the sediment will have settled at the bottom and the water will have a light brown appearance.
3. Pour the brown trifala water into another cup, leaving the sediment in the glass. Save the sediment.
4. Add raw honey (to taste) to the trifala water to make it palatable for a child.
5. Repeat this process by pouring another cup of water into the glass with the same sediment or a new teaspoon of trifala powder. Let it sit all day and have the child drink it (with raw honey as desired) again in the evening.
6. Prepare for the following day by putting a fresh teaspoon of trifala powder in a glass of water to sit overnight.

Castor Oil

Remember that when children are under stress, one of the first places they react is in the digestive system. Although winter kid-types are much more susceptible to becoming constipated due to their tendency toward dryness, any kid-type can become constipated. Since kids may not volunteer details about what happens in the bathroom, it is important for parents to monitor the eliminative habits of their children.

> When my children were young, I noticed that if their elimination was regular, then their chance of avoiding colds was greatly improved.

Recently I noticed that my 7-year-old was taking much longer to go to the bathroom than was usual. This was easy to notice, since, like clockwork, he always has to use the bathroom during a meal at a restaurant. When I found myself waiting for ten minutes in the bathroom for him to finish while my food was getting cold, I became highly motivated to treat his early-stage constipation. This is an example of an easy-to-identify behavioral change revealing the early signs of an imbalance. It is much easier to treat your child at this stage than later, when they have symptoms of a tummyache, cold, flu, or allergy.

Many of us may remember our grandparents giving us teaspoon-sized doses of castor oil (against our will) to make us somehow healthier. This habit still exists in Europe, Asia, and many other parts of the world where traditional medicinal habits prevail. In order for parents to give children things like castor oil, or other untastey concoctions, we may have to get creative.

Although I have heard that some health-food stores are not recommending castor oil for internal consumption, it has been used internally in Ayurveda, safely, for thousands of years. Castor beans—from which the oil is pressed—are poisonous, but when processed, the toxic compounds are removed from the oil. The U.S. Pharmacopoeia lists castor oil as a compound safe for internal consumption, and the U.S. National Institutes of Health label castor oil as a compound that is generally safe.

Castor oil can have a strong laxative effect. I suggest that it be used carefully in small amounts to create gentle bowel movements.

Squirt-Squirt

"Squirt-squirt" is a technique I developed with my children and used with them when they were young. I would pretend that I was a mommy bird and they were baby birds (they absolutely loved to play this game). I had an eyedropper filled with castor oil and some grape juice ready for the "baby birds" to wash down the taste of the oil. I told the kids to line up so I could feed them like birds and then I would squirt a dropper or two full of oil into their open mouths.

I would never give them so much castor oil that it produced a laxative effect; it was just enough to help facilitate a more efficient downwards elimination. If they did have some loose movements as a result of the "squirt-squirt," that meant that I had given them too much. I usually gave only one or two droppers-full of oil; sometimes when they begged for a third, it would usually be just fine. I would make sure to keep an eye on their elimination for the next few hours. If you do decide to try to "squirt-squirt" in your own home, I would recommend getting your children acquainted with it on the weekends when they will be home for a few hours to make sure they are not extra-sensitive to castor oil. This use of castor oil is not recommended for children with loose bowel movements.

This was one of my earlier techniques to prevent colds that worked incredibly well and proved to me time and again that complete and efficient elimination is the key to a healthy child. I have since improved upon this technique and now use a kinder and gentler approach to accomplish the same thing. Plus, my kids soon caught on and realized that "squirt-squirt" was a good time to get out of the kitchen—and quick!

Castor Oil Cookie

A kinder and gentler approach is the "Castor Oil Cookie." Cookies are helpful for children who have chronically slow digestive systems. The recipe calls for about 1 teaspoon of castor oil per cookie, and like "squirt-squirt," it is not enough oil to create a strong laxative effect. If a laxative effect occurs (which means the stools become loose), then reduce the amount of castor oil until the bowel movements are normal. Both the "squirt-squirt" and the cookie, if used at the right dosage, will not cause the stool to become loose. They will actually make the bowel movements more complete while remaining firm. If the stool does become loose, then lower the dose.

 Caution: This recipe is not indicated for children who have loose bowel movements.

List of ingredients:

- Whole wheat flour (about 1/4 cup)
- Water

- Raw sugar or other sweetener (except honey)
- Oil for sautéing

To make castor oil cookies:

1. Take a handful (about 1/4 cup) of whole wheat flour and add enough water to make dough that is light and moist, but not too wet. Start with about half as much water as flour. The exact amount of water needed will vary, depending on factors like humidity.
2. While mixing, slowly add more water as needed. Be careful not to over-mix the flour and water.
3. Add 1 teaspoon of castor oil and 2 teaspoons of raw sugar or other natural sweetener (Sucanat, maple syrup, or stevia, but not honey).
4. Either sauté the mixture in hot oil (olive oil, or any good-quality cooking oil) like a pancake, or a shape it into a flat ball and bake it in a preheated oven (375°F) for 10 to 12 minutes, like a cookie.

Eat one cookie daily for several weeks (three months at the most) to restore proper elimination. Make the cookie fresh daily. (It only takes a few minutes to prepare.)

Castor oil used in this recipe is different from standard laxatives for two reasons. First, the amount of castor oil used in the cookie is not a dose that is irritating to the bowel. Secondly, castor oil is an amazing lubricant. In fact, during World War I, it was the lubricant of choice for 12-cylinder airplane engines. While most laxatives are astringent and drying in nature, causing them to irritate the intestinal wall, the lubricating effect of castor oil restores the natural balance of the intestinal environment. The intestines require an slightly oily environment for healthy bacteria to flourish and to maintain the contractility of the intestinal wall. This is one of the reasons that low-fat or no-fat diets are seldom recommended in Ayurveda, and why the notion that fat is bad is a big mistake for a child's perfect health. (We will visit this subject in Chapters 6 and 7.)

Asafoetida/Hing

When digestion and elimination are slow, the intestines can become toxic as the stagnant food putrefies and ferments inside the gut, causing gas and bloating. Gas buildup is a common cause of stomachaches in kids, for which there are some very simple remedies. Asafoetida (sometimes called hing) is one of these; it is a pungent herb which is a gas- and mucus-reducing herb for the digestive tract.

- Its botanical name is *Ferula asafoetida.*
- Hing helps to strengthen the digestive fire while it simultaneously removes excess mucus and accumulated gas, and decreases bloating.
- Use hing for flatulence, indigestion, intestinal cramping, abdominal pain, and constipation.
- It is commonly used as a spice to add flavor and reduce gas-producing potential of foods like beans and lentils. A pinch or 1/4 teaspoon is usually enough since hing is very strong.
- Hing is highly effective for impacted fecal matter and severe constipation. It pulls the assimilation-compromising hardened mucus off the intestinal lining.

How To Take Hing

When taken as a single herb, the dose used is small: 100–200 milligrams of powder with warm water before each meal. It can be taken in capsules or as a powder mixed into a paste with raw honey to make it more palatable.

Hing can be mixed with trikatu if the digestion seems very slow and the symptoms of indigestion are worse after eating a heavy or cheesy meal. Usually 1/2 teaspoon of hing with 1/4 teaspoon of trikatu mixed with raw honey into a paste is a great pre-meal cocktail. Children should take 1/2 teaspoon of this mixture before meals.

Hing can be mixed with trifala if there is constipation along with chronic gas and bloating. If this is indicated, you'll often see a heavy, thick, white coating covering the back of the tongue. Within a week or so of taking the hing and trifala mixture, the white coating on the tongue should start to disappear, and the symptoms of constipation and gas should steadily diminish. To take, mix equal parts of each herb with raw honey into a paste and eat 1/2 to 1 teaspoon either before or after meals. Take this mixture with a large glass of room-temperature water.

To make cumin-ginger tea for gas and bloating:

1. Mix 1/3 teaspoon of powdered cumin with 2/3 teaspoon powdered ginger in 1 1/2 cups of water on the stove.
2. Boil the mixture down to one-half the starting volume (3/4 cup).
3. Add a pinch of sea salt, a few drops of lemon juice, and some raw honey to taste.

How To Take Cumin-Ginger Tea

Have your child sip the warm tea either before meals or on an empty stomach.

To increase the potency of this tea, use cumin seeds instead of powdered cumin and heat 1/3 teaspoon of the seeds in a dry pan without oil. Then grind the seeds into a powder and follow previous directions.

Zach

In extreme cases, constipation caused by a drying out of the mucous membranes can alternate with chronic diarrhea. These situations require us to remove the excess mucus, heal the mucous membranes, and reset the ability of the upper digestive system to properly break down food and prepare it for absorption and elimination.

Zach was a 7-year-old boy who came to my office complaining of loose bowel movements, chronic colds, and breathing difficulties. He had a history of frequent constipation and chronic colds over the past few years. The chronicity of these complaints had caused all of his mucous membranes to be inflamed and irritated. He was a winter kid-type with dry skin and some minor lingering skin rashes.

Treating a boy like Zach is challenging because there are only a limited number of herbal remedies that this overly irritated system can handle. If I were to overwhelm him by trying to treat too many things at once, he would resist everything and we would make no progress. In his case, my first concern was to heal and repair the irritated mucous membranes.

The one herb that would best address all of his conditions is turmeric. With such an intense inflammation, Zach's body needed a natural anti-inflammatory substance. Turmeric is the most powerful non-steroidal anti-inflammatory on the market. It treats irritation in the sinuses, respiratory and intestinal tracts, and skin, and it is indicated for diarrhea. To reduce the inflammation and to heal and repair the tissues in Zach's mucous membranes, I asked his mom to give him 1 teaspoon of turmeric as a paste with honey between three and six times a day for seven days. Within three days of taking turmeric, Zach's diarrhea was relieved and his cold improved.

As I treated him, I had to be sure the constipation that preceded his current complaint of chronic loose movements was not reactivated. To prevent this, I recommended that Zach's parents pay attention to his bowel regularity and have some trifala on hand to use as needed to keep his elimination regular. I asked Zach to take one or two tablets of trifala before bed and in the morning as needed to maintain normal elimination, once the course of turmeric was complete.

Diarrhea

There are many natural remedies that are effective for treating loose bowel movements in children. The herbs typically used have an astringent effect that assists in the absorption of excess liquid from the stool. Using turmeric as an initial treatment, as I did with Zach, helps to calm the irritated mucosa. Once the chronic inflammation is arrested, the commonly used herbs to treat diarrhea will be more effective.

The following list contains remedies for diarrhea:

- Natural blackberry juice or fresh blackberries
- Stewed apples
- Tapioca pudding
- Arrowroot (as a thickener in sauces and desserts)
- Pomegranates or pomegranate juice
- Nutmeg

Another remedy for loose movements is to remove the seeds of a pomegranate and grind the remainder (the rind and septum) into a paste with a mortar and pestle. Take 1 teaspoon of the paste four times a day. Dried septum and rind can be ground into a powder and saved for future use.

Nutmeg is a common household spice that is one of the most potent herbs for increasing absorption in the small intestine and for treating diarrhea.

A classic remedy to stop diarrhea is to drink warm buttermilk with 250–500 milligrams of nutmeg added in.

Small amounts of nutmeg can also be mixed with other digestive herbs, such as ginger and cumin, to enhance the absorption of food through the small intestine. These medicinal herbs can also be used simply as spices and added to foods while cooking.

Caution: You can have too much of a good thing with nutmeg. Taking more than 3 teaspoons of nutmeg per day can make a child (or an adult) sick.

To prevent dehydration during bouts of diarrhea, take plenty of fluids, especially warm water. To replace lost, use an electrolyte replacement drink. The most natural one I have seen is Knuden's Recharge.

You can also use the following homemade mixture:

1. Combine the juice of two limes or lemons (not too sour) with 3 cups of water.

2. Add 1 teaspoon of salt (it should not be too salty).
3. Add 1/2 cup of sugar (it should be sweet but not too heavy).
4. Place the mixture with ice in an insulated bottle and drink throughout the day.

Soup To Improve Digestion and Cure Colds

The following recipe is for a soup that is easy to digest and can be eaten at any time of the year by any kid-type. Not only are many illnesses in children caused by weak or sluggish digestion, but when children are sick, the strength of their digestion becomes significantly reduced, affecting the absorption of nutrients. Chronic loose bowel movements are another cause of dehydration and mineral and nutrient deficiencies.

This soup recipe is a medicinal treatment for digestive difficulties like gas, malabsorption of food, and general weakness. It is safe and beneficial for babies, pregnant women, the elderly, and everyone in between. It is a perfect source of easy-to-digest proteins that are needed to help a child recover from a cold, flu, or stomach virus.

Ingredients:

1 cup split yellow mung beans (found in health food stores and Asian, Middle Eastern, or Indian food stores)
2 cups white basmati rice
1 inch fresh ginger root, chopped
1 small handful of fresh cilantro leaves, chopped
2 tablespoons of ghee (clarified butter)
1 teaspoon turmeric
1 teaspoon coriander powder
1 teaspoon cumin powder
1 teaspoon whole cumin seeds
1 teaspoon mustard seeds
1 teaspoon kosher or rock salt
1 pinch of hing or asafoetida
7–10 cups of water
Bragg Liquid Aminos (optional: for flavor or salt substitute)

To make the soup:

1. Rinse beans and rice together until the water runs clear.
2. In a large pot on medium heat mix: ghee, mustard seeds, turmeric, hing, ginger, cumin seeds, and cumin and coriander powder. Stir together for a few minutes, lightly sautéing the spices.
3. Add rice and beans and stir again until they are coated with the spices and ghee.
4. Add the water and salt and bring to a boil.
5. Boil for 10 minutes.
6. Reduce the heat to low, cover the pot, and continue to cook until rice and beans become soft. (about 30 to 40 minutes)
7. Add the cilantro leaves (and optional liquid aminos) just before serving.

Trifala and Bilva

When I come across a case of diarrhea that is not responding to the standard diarrhea treatments, I use a combination of trifala and an herb called *bilva*. Bilva's botanical name is *Agele marmelos*. It is astringent, pungent, and bitter. Bilva is the most effective herb for pulling chronic mucus off the small and large intestines and stopping diarrhea naturally.

How To Take Trifala and Bilva

I typically recommend using 1/2 teaspoon of trifala and 1/2 teaspoon of bilva with warm water after meals or on an empty stomach. They can be taken as a paste with raw honey, in capsules, or mixed with water.

Using these herbs together is not only an extremely effective treatment for diarrhea; it also truly addresses the cause of the problem. In this case, the cause is chronic obstructive mucus causing constipation and diarrhea as well as chronic malabsorption (interference with the digestive system's ability to properly absorb food).

Summer Kid-Type Digestion

Summer kid-types tend to be more aggressive and competitive, and they often have very strong digestive systems. They dislike hot weather and they don't have a strong affinity for sunbathing because they already have a surplus of internal heat. When out of balance, their stomachs tend to produce excess acidity and heat. This heat can irritate and inflame both the stomach lining and the intestinal wall. As with the other kid-types, excess mucus is often produced by the stomach and intestines, in this case as a protection against the chronic irritation.

Unfortunately, children do not usually notice the excess heat and inflammation building up in their intestinal tracts. When these kid-types reach adulthood, they may complain of symptoms such as heartburn and colitis. More often than not, neither summer kid-types nor their parents will notice the inflammation until symptoms appear elsewhere throughout the body. These symptoms may include: skin rashes, acne, allergies, and diarrhea (see diarrhea treatments starting on page 94).

When the unbalanced summer kid-type's digestive system cannot effectively eliminate wastes, the circulatory system carries the excess heat throughout the body, searching for a means of elimination.

The heat, acidity, and toxins are carried through the circulatory system in an attempt to eliminate them through the skin. As the summer kid-types try to eliminate toxins through the skin, they are prone to developing rashes, hives, or acne. To properly address skin and circulatory issues, we must first reduce the heat and inflammation in the digestive system so that it can eliminate toxins more effectively.

> Summer kid-types tend to have a sensitive circulatory system in the same way that winter kid-types have sensitive nervous systems and spring kid-types tend to retain water and become congested.

Fennel-Coriander Tea

One of the most cooling and soothing herbal remedies to balance summer-type digestion is fennel-coriander tea.

To make fennel-coriander tea:

> Add 2 teaspoons of fennel seeds and 2 teaspoons of coriander seeds to 1 quart of water and boil for 5 minutes (for a weak tea) or 10 minutes (for a strong tea).

How To Take Fennel-Coriander Tea

The tea can be taken hot, with sweetener as desired. Summer kid-types can also drink this tea cool or at room temperature throughout the day. It also goes well with meals, as it stimulates digestion while cooling an overheated intestinal tract.

It is especially useful in the summer months to cool summer kid-types who are less tolerant of the heat.

When fennel is used alone in a tea, it is excellent for strengthening weak digestion in all kid-types. Adding coriander gives the tea a more cooling action.

No Waste Out

While summer kid-types rarely complain of constipation, that does not necessarily mean that their digestion and assimilation is optimal. The out-of-balance digestive system of a summer kid-type has a tendency to become too hot and acidic. When excess inflammation and acidity in an overheated summer kid-type causes reactive mucus production, the excess mucus lining the intestinal wall compromises the absorption of nutrients and allows wastes and impurities to enter the body's circulation.

Think of a dirty air filter—the dirtier it gets, the less it cleans the air moving through it, allowing impure air to be recirculated. In the same way, when the intestines are lined with a layer of excess mucus, impurities will be recirculated into the blood and lymphatic systems. This area is especially vulnerable to the dirty-filter effect; about half of the intestinal area is drained by the blood stream, and the other half is drained by the lymphatic system, which provides ample opportunity for the reabsorbtion of toxic material. The reabsorbtion and recirculation of toxic material in the body is dangerous because once these impurities reach the blood stream or lymphatic system, the body reabsorbs toxins through the portal system into the liver. So these toxins first impact the liver, and ultimately the skin.

Over time this reabsorbtion of toxins can cause a host of imbalances in your child. Summer kid-types, with their sensitive circulatory systems, are especially prone to react to a buildup of impurities in the blood or lymphatic fluid. The accumulation of toxins can cause skin rashes, allergies, asthma, food intolerance, acne, fatigue, and the inability to concentrate.

Summer Circulation

There are two very important remedies to improve the circulatory system and remove accumulated toxins in summer kid-types. One remedy, manjistha, is specific for the lymphatic system; the other, neem, purifies the blood, liver, and skin. Both remedies treat the symptoms that show up on the skin by eliminating toxins from the body's fluids—thus treating the cause of these symptoms.

Neem to the Rescue

Neem is an extremely beneficial herb that helps to cleanse and detoxify the blood, liver, and skin.

Neem's botanical name is *Azadirachta indica.* The bark and leaves of this large and common tropical deciduous tree are used for their bitter and cooling properties. Neem is the most powerful herb for treating and curing skin diseases, fevers, and skin rashes.

How To Take Neem

The leaves can be made into a tea and used topically on skin rashes and inflammation. The powdered leaves can be used internally in a capsule to purify the blood and skin.

The recommended internal dose is 250–500 milligrams of the

powdered herb after each meal. It needs to be taken for between one and three months to root out impurities deep within the tissues that can be the underlying cause of acne and other hard-to-treat skin irritations.

Neem is very cooling, so be careful not to give neem if your child is complaining of being cold.

Manjistha and Lymphatic Drainage

The Forgotten Lymph

I have mentioned the lymphatic system several times. This is because it is one of the most important systems of the body—the home of the immune system. When the lymphatic system becomes stagnant, the immune system also slows down. In a slow lymphatic system, the circulating immune cells become stuck, like a fire engine blocked by a traffic jam, unable to reach its destination.

The lymphatic system can become sluggish not only through boggy digestion and buildup of toxins, but also through a sedentary lifestyle. Unlike the bloodstream, the lymphatic fluid is not pumped by the heart's beating. Rather, muscular contractions move the lymphatic fluid through the body. One of the important benefits of exercise (discussed in Chapter 11) is the enhanced circulation of lymphatic fluid. Anything that compromises lymphatic flow can disrupt the movement of the white blood cells and therefore impair the immune system's ability to flush toxins from the tissues. When the lymphatic system is unable to remove waste efficiently, it dumps the impurities into muscles, joints, skin, and other tissues of the body.

One of the most common recipients of this waste material is the skin, which is why skin conditions appear as a result of poor digestion or lymphatic congestion, especially in summer kid-types. The joints are another vulnerable area of the body that end up becoming a repository for toxins the body is unable to eliminate. Joint problems seldom appear in children, but the seeds for adult joint problems are sown in poor digestion and compromised lymphatic flow when young.

Allergies are also linked to digestion, skin conditions, and lymphatic flow. When the lymphatic system cannot remove waste, the body can become hypersensitive to hard-to-digest foods, pollutants, and pollens, causing severe and even chronic allergic reactions. Again, we see that the causes of many allergic reactions and skin conditions have their roots in digestive and circulatory problems. Neem assists in detoxifying the skin, but if the skin cannot drain properly through the lymphatic fluid, it will remain toxic. In many cases, neem can be used with manjistha, an herb that is well known as a blood, lymph, and skin cleanser. Manjistha was first introduced in Chapter 3.

Manjistha

Manjistha removes obstructions in the blood and lymph and is traditionally used for tumors and stones.

Manjistha has such profound healing properties that it is used to help repair broken bones. It does so by improving the drainage of the lymphatic system, thus dramatically improving the body's healing abilities. The key to healing any aspect of the human body is blood flow; if lymphatic fluid cannot drain properly, new blood is unable to flow into the area of the body needing repair.

How To Take Manjistha

Manjistha is a cooling herb and can be used topically for skin rashes or skin discolorations. Make a paste by mixing the powered herb with honey and applying it to the skin lesion.

Manjistha can also be taken orally; the usual dose for a child is 300–500 milligrams, two or three times a day with water, after meals or on an empty stomach.

When To Use Manjistha:

Some of the most common symptoms of lymphatic congestion and indications for using manjistha are:

- Swollen, puffy eyes, hands, and feet

- Skin rashes
- Fatigue
- Allergies
- Aching in joints that moves from one place to another
- Sore throats
- Acne
- Itchy skin that gets worse with exercise

A Final Word on Digestion

It is the things we do every day of our lives, day in and day out, that can be the most debilitating or rejuvenating for our bodies. If our lifestyle habits are inconsistent and stressful, our bodies are sure to break down prematurely. On the other hand, if we cultivate good habits and a regular routine, no matter what the routine is, our bodies stand a good chance of maintaining perfect health throughout our lives.

There are a few important rules to follow to support the digestive system that are typically unheard of in our American diet and way of life. I do not expect that every child and parent will follow these tips to support good digestion, but it is important for families and children to move in this direction and understand these rules.

Have the attitude that these are suggestions to aspire to rather than rigid rules you must adhere to.

Code of Digestive Intelligence

- Eat in a settled atmosphere.
- Sit down to eat (sitting in a car doesn't count).
- Eat only when hungry.
- Favor freshly prepared foods.
- Avoid ice-cold food and drinks (particularly in the winter).
- Eat at a moderate pace—don't eat too slowly or too quickly.
- Eat only if previous meal is digested, usually after a minimum of one hour.
- Take a few sips of water with meals.
- Include cooked foods in meals, they are easier to digest.

- Sit quietly for a few minutes after eating.
- Make eating an enjoyable experience that you look forward to.
- Close the kitchen as early in the evening as possible.
- Make the midday meal the largest meal of the day.
- If you overeat at lunch, rest for ten minutes lying down on your left side.

Things to avoid:

- Don't drink milk with meals.
- Don't heat or cook with honey.
- Don't talk while chewing.
- Never eat when upset.
- Don't watch TV, read, open mail, or talk on the phone while eating.
- And most of all—don't stand up while eating.

> There is an old Vedic saying: If you eat standing up, death looks over your shoulder.

Chapter 5

Secret 4—The Fountain of Youth

once de León, the sixteenth-century Spanish explorer, spent his life searching for what he called the Fountain of Youth. Today, the modern search for the fountain of youth, or the elixir of life, continues with contemporary life-extension specialists (such as Dr. Bernard Jensen) who have researched the diets and habits of people from cultures around the world who have lived to well over 100 years. Research by Dr. Jensen and others clearly shows that a pure and simple lifestyle, with a source of pure water and natural eating habits connected to the local farmer, are major factors in the life-extension equation.

Unlike Americans, who exist on a standard diet rich in processed and packaged foods, long-lived populations around the world have sustained themselves with a diet devoid of our modern conveniences. Foods were once chosen from the harvests of the season and cooked fresh daily. Current research confirms that the *quality* of food is part of the elixir of life we search for. The health-giving benefits of this ancient and successful approach to food can easily be incorporated into a modern kid-friendly lifestyle (discussed in Chapter 7).

Food is not the only component of living a long and healthy life. Ponce de León was onto something when he was looking for a mythical fountain. Probably the most frequently recurring theme in the field of life-extension research is that water is the catalyst for a longer and healthier life. In this chapter, I will discuss a simple and profound healing secret: the importance of drinking pure water and staying properly hydrated. Unfortunately, this practice has almost disappeared in today's American culture.

A recent report noted that 70% of pre-school children drank no pure water. This is partly because parents have gotten it into their heads that children should drink juice, and seldom offer water. Children are creatures of habit—if you feed them water at a young age, they will become water-drinkers. But if you feed them juice and soda, this habit will lead them to become dehydrated over time, making them more susceptible to illness. Drinking the right amount of the purest water available can be your child's best medicine.

 Secret 4: The fourth secret to health is drinking enough pure water to stay fully hydrated. This practice supports the immune system, increases strength and vitality, improves physical and athletic performance, and decreases your child's susceptibility to getting sick.

Around the world, certain waters have been heralded as healing waters or fountains of youth and still attract thousands of believers. Most of these accolades are founded on folklore rather than science. However, it should be well understood that not all waters are created equal. Some types of water hydrate the body more effectively than others. Being properly hydrated can be powerful medicine. In our society, where we drink more soft drinks than water, our children's perfect health may depend on us remembering the power of the mythical Fountain of Youth.

Lack of proper hydration is beginning to be looked at by Western medicine as a potential cause for many of the chronic diseases we experience. According to a Cornell University study, some of the early signs that dehydration has begun are dry skin, headaches, and fatigue. The insidious onset of chronic, severe dehydration can cause blood pressure and circulatory concerns, digestive difficulties, kidney dysfunction and severe problems in just about any system of the body. That same study revealed that the majority of Americans may be suffering from some degree of dehydration. Let's examine the role water plays in maintaining a healthy body.

When we are born, our bodies are made up of 78% water. We all know how supple and soft the skin of babies can be—they bend and twist while staying plump like a water balloon. The level of elasticity that we see in infants and small children does not have to disappear, but, unfortunately, it does. According to the water bottling company, Penta Water, studies have shown that by the time we are between 50 and 60 years old, the body is only 50% water. Slowly, over time, we lose our elasticity and become more brittle.

This water loss occurs over time as a result of chronic and long-standing dehydration. When we are born, most of the water in our bodies is inside the membranes of cells, making the cells themselves vital and robust. As we age and dehydrate, these water-based intracellular fluids leave the cell, collect in the spaces between cells, and then become unable to reenter the cell. There are many reasons why the extra-cellular water has difficulty reentering the cell membrane and rejuvenating cellular function as we age. Some of the factors affecting this process are stress, lack of adequate oxygen and blood supply to the cells, dehydration, impure water, coffee, soda pop, and alcohol. Each of them plays a part in the chronic dehydration of the body and the premature aging process.

Just Water

Water is known chemically as H_2O, signifying that each molecule of water is made up of one oxygen and two hydrogen atoms. The water molecule is known as a polar molecule, which means that it is not neutral, but has a slight electrical charge to it. This charge attracts other polar substances to it, making it sticky by nature. Other electrically charged polar substances include: salts, sugars, vinegar, many of the flavorings in food, and alcohol. These are substances that can dissolve in water. Oils are non-polar, meaning they contain no electrical charge and are thus unable to dissolve in water or mix with it at all. Thus the expression "they go together like oil and water," meaning that they don't go together, because no matter how hard you shake a bottle containing these two liquids, they will not mix together and will always separate again.

The nature of the water molecule is to be sticky. It attracts anything and everything (with an electrical charge). The affinity water has for making solutions is the reason that we can make instant tea, lemonade, or orange juice. This property of water makes it an amazing solvent in the body and allows the substances of the cell to be contained within it. But water's stickiness can make it cumbersome as it attracts salts, minerals, or other substances. Water naturally passes in and out of cells through specialized hydration channels in the cell membrane called aquaporins. But when the water has a collection of materials stuck to it, the molecules become unwieldy and too large to fit through the small aquaporins, which are designed exclusively for H_2O.

Most of the water we drink is loaded down with dissolved solids like minerals, heavy metals, sugars, or chemicals that make hydrating a cell like trying to get into a phone booth with twenty backpacks on. The water is passing over the cells and simply not hydrating them. This is why when people drink lots and lots of water they feel like "it goes right through them." They still feel thirsty, and they find themselves frequenting the bathroom as the water literally passes right through them after it passes over all their cells. Water quality is what determines whether the water penetrates the cells and maintains optimal cellular function or just passes over the cells, escorting you to the bathroom.

There are many varieties of water—and some are better than others. Unfortunately for our kids' health, most of them drink an assortment of beverages other than water. Before we examine different types of water, let's take a look at some dehydrating beverages.

While fruit juices, instant Kool-Aid, or other drink mixes are not in the category of *really* dehydrating beverages, they will not contribute to the amount of pure water needed to properly hydrate the body. As previously mentioned, water will attract any electrically charged molecule to it. The water molecule must shed these hitchhikers before it is able to enter the aquaporins and hydrate the cell. If certain dissolved solids are not digested or stripped from the water molecule, then the water runs over the cell's surface like water off a duck's back, sliding over the feathers and not wetting its skin.

Water is also necessary to digest and break down sugars and proteins. This is one of the reasons that it is important to drink *pure* water. When we drink milk or juices, some of the water or fluid they contain is used to digest the sugars and proteins in the drink.

Juices are able to offer the body a certain level of hydration, but they can sometimes do more harm than good. Many juices you buy at the store have more concentrated sugar or high-fructose corn syrup than pure juice. These concentrated sugars dramatically affect blood sugar levels, and ultimately energy level and mood. Fluctuations in blood sugar and resultant stress negatively impact the circulatory system, fat metabolism, cholesterol levels, fat metabolism, and the ability of the body to bring both vital nutrition and water to the deep tissues.

High-fructose corn syrup, the super-sweet sweetener found in most juice drinks and soda pops, was introduced to America in 1970, conspicuously when child obesity levels began to soar. It is linked directly to increased triglyceride levels. In fact, studies show that high-fructose corn syrup is directly converted to triglycerides rather than glucose, which is the brain's fuel supply. High-fructose corn syrup has also been linked to increased levels of obesity and may be a poor source of energy in the body since it is not converted to glucose as other carbohydrates are.

In order to hydrate your children and wean them off sugary or super-sweet, non-hydrating drinks, it is necessary to get them to drink more water. To get them used to the taste of drinks that are not sugary and sweet, dilute fruit juices with water and choose juices that do not have added sugar. Slowly introduce pure water into their diet. One way to do this is to give them a bottle of water—rather than a juice box—with their school lunch. Make a glass of water a mandatory drink with breakfast and after school.

Let's Talk Soda Pop

In 1850, Americans drank about 13 ounces of soda pop per year. Today, according to the National Soft Drink Association, Americans consume more soft drinks than they do water. In fact, for every 16 ounces of bottled water consumed, Americans drank 64 ounces of soda pop. The average 12- to 19-year-old soda pop-consuming male drinks more than two cans per day, or 868 cans annually. This is a significant amount of soda. When we consider the fact that kids are drinking such large amounts of soda pop, we should know exactly what it's comprised of. One 20-ounce can of cola contains: carbonated water, natural and artificial flavors, caffeine, and 17 teaspoons of sugar. Each 12-ounce can packs a 250-calorie caffeinated jolt to your child's nervous system. According to a study published in the November 2002 *Journal of the American Medical Association,* 24% of adolescents drank at least 26 ounces of soda pop each day. According to the Beverage Marketing Corporation, more than 9 billion gallons, on average, are consumed each year.

The top five soda pops are:

1. **Coca-Cola Classic**—3.1 billion gallons
2. **Pepsi**—2.2 billion gallons
3. **Diet Coke**—1.3 billion gallons
4. **Mountain Dew**—1 billion gallons
5. **Sprite**—992 million gallons

These soda pops are so saturated with sugars, flavors, and preservatives that they are far from able to hydrate the body at a cellular level. This solution is just too clumpy to even attempt to squeeze through the water-selective aquaporins. Adding to soda's dehydrating effect, caffeine is a known diuretic (it increases urine output so more water is lost in urine), so sodas containing caffeine cause more fluid loss than fluid absorption into the body. The astringent taste of most soft drinks amplifies this effect. Non-caffeinated soft drinks are less dehydrating to the body, but still do not provide a significant hydrating benefit because of the stickiness of the sugar solution to the water molecules.

Soft drink consumption is big business in the United States, and so is dehydration. According to the National Soft Drink Association of America, Americans spend $60 billion on soft drinks each year. Every day, the major soft drink companies do their best to convince us to buy and drink soda pop—the Coca-Cola and Pepsi companies alone spend close to $3 billion in advertising per year. Overall, Americans are consuming twice as much soda pop as they did 25 years ago—and they're spending $60 billion a year on it. That's twice the amount that Americans spend on books.

Soft drink companies don't stop at advertising to sell their products to our children. At the present time, 60% of all American middle schools and high schools are selling soda pop in vending machines. What's even worse is that, according to *the Journal of the American Medical Association,* 240 school districts have signed exclusive contracts with beverage companies for "pouring rights," meaning that a school enters into an exclusive relationship with a beverage company to have its vending machines in hallways and cafeterias. The beverage companies contract to have their logos appear on scoreboards, in hallways, and on book covers. Some school districts have received signing bonuses of more than $1 million to promote soft drink products. Many of these contracts reward schools with sales bonuses for high volumes of sales.

The volume of soft drinks consumed in schools is astonishing. In the Los Angeles Unified School District, $4.5 million worth of soft drinks were sold to students in the year 2000. A major loss in revenue to soda pop companies occurred when both the Los Angeles and Oakland, California, school districts later banned the sale of soft drinks in their schools in an effort to protect their students' health.

There is currently an active debate about health risks posed by children's consumption of soft drinks. Aside from the debate, one has to ask what the motivation could be for enticing school children to drink caffeinated soda pops as a regular beverage in schools. The health benefits don't seem to be at the top of the list. As for health risks, how many parents would feed their children 17 teaspoons of

> **Consumption of soft drinks affects both boys and girls. Between 40% and 60% of the body's peak bone mass is built during the teenage years.**

refined sugar in one sitting—and repeat that several times each day in the name of good health?

One of the areas in which the negative consequences of drinking soda pop (especially for children and teenagers) is currently being studied is the effect that drinking phosphoric acid-containing sodas (primarily cola drinks) has on the development of proper bone density through the deposition of calcium in the bones. Phosphoric acid interferes with the body's ability to absorb and metabolize calcium, and excessive phosphorous intake causes the body to leach calcium from the bones. The teen years are the most important time for the body to lay down bone density, and the development of osteoporosis later in life is linked to the strength of bone health in childhood and young adulthood. Limiting ingestion of cola drinks is recommended to build healthy bones for life. A 2002 review in *Adolescent Medicine* discusses this issue. But it is not only future bone structure that is affected by too much soda. Research done by Harvard University following 460 ninth- and tenth-grade girls showed a link between consumption of soda pop, especially cola drinks, and higher risk of bone fractures.

> A questionnaire was given to 460 girls in the ninth and tenth grades, asking them about their diet and exercise habits, along with any history of bone fractures. The study results showed that girls who drank soft drinks were more than three times more likely to have had a bone fracture. Physically active girls who drank cola drinks were nearly five times more likely to have had a bone fracture.

> Phosphoric acid is detrimental to bone health; its acidic nature causes the body to pull minerals such as calcium out of the bones in order to buffer the acid.

The Can or the Couch

Probably the biggest health concern with regard to soda pop is the extremely high obesity rate we see in children today. *The New York Times* reported in 2002 that more than one billion people worldwide are overweight or obese. In the United States, 64.5% of adults and 15% of children are overweight, with the greatest increase in numbers having occurred in the past 10 years. Clearly, the rising obesity levels in children cannot be blamed only on our increasing soft drink consumption. Lack of activity and a poor overall diet are also major contributors.

The California Center for Public Health Advocacy analyzed the 2001 California Physical Fitness Tests of fifth-, seventh-, and ninth-graders. Results showed that among all students in the 57th Assembly District:

- 32.4% of children were overweight—among the highest%ages in the state.
- 41% of children were unfit.
- The *Journal of the American Medical Association* reported in 1998 that only 1% of children regularly ate diets conforming to the recommendations of the Food Guide Pyramid and 45% failed to achieve *any* of the Pyramid recommendations.
- In 1991, 11 million children between the ages of 6 and 17 were overweight, and 50% did not get enough exercise to develop healthy hearts and lungs.
- According to the standards of the U. S. Amateur Athletic Association, 68% of kids between the ages of 6 and 17 have below-average cardiovascular fitness, flexibility, and abdominal and upper body strength. This has decreased 11% since 1981.
- Health risks from obesity have recently been upgraded in a Rand Co. research report; they are now worse than the health risks from smoking, drinking, and poverty.

Aside from American kids being out of shape and sedentary, the effects of drinking calorie-rich and nutrient-poor soda pop still can't be ignored in the fight against obesity. Melinda Sothern, Ph.D., the co-author of *Trim Kids,* has found that many of the severely obese kids who visit her weight-loss clinic "drink their calories." One 9-year-old girl weighing over 300 pounds recently visited the clinic accompanied by her perplexed mother. The mother couldn't understand why her daughter was so large—after all, she didn't eat much. When questioned by the staff, the girl reported that she drank four or five 20-ounce sodas a day. This daily intake of about 1,000 to 1,250 nutrient-free calories is a prescription for packing on the pounds!

Even though many people argue that soft drinks do not contribute to weight gain and should not be targeted as "the cause," I disagree. If kids drank soda in moderation and corporations didn't spend billions of dollars in marketing efforts aimed at kids, then soda might be a harmless and occasional treat for kids and water would still be the routine drink of choice.

There is strong evidence that many of those liquid calories do turn to fat. In a study that was the first of its kind, Harvard researchers tracked both the weights and the soft drink consumption of 548 grade-school children for two years. As reported in the February 17, 2001, issue of *Lancet,* each daily serving of a sugary drink appears to raise the risk of obesity by 60%.

When it comes to giving soda pop to children, parents need to use common sense. If the average teenager drinks two 12-ounce cans of soda pop each day, he or she might as well be eating 24 teaspoons of white refined sugar. If the drink is caffeinated, then it not only negatively impacts blood sugar, moods, and energy levels, but it is also an energy-robbing stimulant (because it stimulates the body's adrenal glands to release stress hormones) and a powerful dehydrating agent.

When it comes to giving your children soda pop, make it a special occasion and not a daily event. The easiest way to do this is to keep soda out of the house—and for parents to act as role models and not drink soda pop daily in front of their kids. This is what we do in our house. Our kids may drink soda pop as a treat while at a restaurant or birthday party, but when at home the drink of choice with meals is water or a natural juice. What's interesting is that I find our kids actually prefer water when they are thirsty. They tend to want soda pop when they are hungry—no doubt they are seeking the 12 teaspoons of easily absorbed sugar.

Some parents may find that they are able to completely eliminate soda pop from their child's diet. In many cases, kids actually lose the taste for soda and don't drink it outside the home even if they have the opportunity. This is a personal choice by both the parent and child, and it is clearly the healthiest decision. The only caveat that I have is to remind parents that if you force an extremely restrictive diet and lifestyle on your children you may provide them with years of motivation to rebel against those very restrictions. But there are many children who will not view the lack of soda as a restriction; they may even think it's cool. This refreshing attitude seems to depend on how the restriction is presented and enforced. In my opinion, there is no right or wrong on this issue, it is mostly a matter of moderation, communication, and awareness of your children's needs.

Diet Soda

Most diet sodas are sweetened with the amino-acid-based artificial sweetener aspartame. This calorie-free sweetener tastes 180 times sweeter than sugar. Aspartame is used not only in soft drinks; it is used in over 5,000 commercially available food products. There has been an on-going controversy about its safety ever since it was introduced in 1980. In the intestinal tract, aspartame is converted into aspartate, phenylalanine, and an alcohol formaldehyde or wood alcohol. The alcohol formaldehyde is a known toxin that is thought to be detoxified and rendered harmless by the liver. Aspartate and phenylalanine are central nervous system stimulants. In fact, aspartate does not have to be modified in any way in order to affect the central nervous system; it uniquely stimulates the brain directly. The question is whether the brain, especially a child's brain, can handle the intense stimulation of such a powerful neurotransmitter. In a world where over-stimulation is chronic, parents should be seeking out ways to reduce their child's stimulation.

But what about drinking diet sodas to encourage weight loss? It is questionable as to whether aspatame has any real benefit in the weight-loss equation. When you drink a diet soda that tastes super-sweet, the taste buds receive a sweet signal, and the aspartame itself stimulates the nervous system. But in a diet soda there are no calories to back up this stimulation. With the sensation of the sweet taste experienced, the body expects some calorie-rich fuel to provide energy. Without it, the brain rebounds from the sweet message by demanding fuel—and feeling hungry and unsatisfied.

This lack of satisfaction can come from excessive use of diet products, so the diet-soda-drinker constantly feels hungry because the body is craving a real meal. This isn't a great formula for long-term weight loss. If a child has a weight problem, give water instead of diet soda. Water will satisfy the child's thirst and will not initiate any short- or long-term lack of satisfaction. It is also possible that dehydration is one of the factors behind the weight problem in the first place, an issue I will address later in this chapter.

Caffeine and Dehydration

Caffeine is one of the dehydrating ingredients found in many flavors and types of soda pop. The caffeine in cola or other soft drinks is an ingredient that is completely added—and comes from the caffeine taken out when coffee is decaffeinated! Caffeine is a diuretic, which means that it causes the body to lose water by stimulating the kidneys to release more water into the urine. Drinking these caffeinated drinks causes you to lose more water than you actually take in, and thus they have a net effect of being dehydrating. Any caffeinated beverage like tea, coffee, or cola is dehydrating because of the diuretic and astringent properties of caffeine.

Alcohol and Dehydration

Caffeine is not the only commonly consumed diuretic. Alcohol is a powerful diuretic; the feeling of a hangover largely results from the dehydrating effect of alcohol on the cells. Since alcohol is made up primarily of sugar, and the brain uses up to 80% of our sugar supply, it is not surprising that the brain is typically the most strongly affected by alcohol and by the dehydrating effect of a hangover. The cells of the nervous system are especially sensitive to changes in the maintenance of their water and electrolyte balance. Although the dehydrating effects of alcohol should not be a concern with young children, alcohol use and abuse can be a concern with teenagers, even with children in their pre-adolescent years. Aside from the host of other issues associated with alcohol, its diuretic effects—even for adults—are a serious concern in the quest to stay fully hydrated.

SUPER-VISION

Restricted diets have been a part of the American appetite for many years now. Each best-selling diet lasts only long enough to be replaced by the next best-selling diet. When adults stop eating certain things because they are known to put on weight, it is only a matter of months before the cravings start. When you restrict certain foods, you will find yourself binging on the very food you decided not to eat. Our children are no different. Instead of restricting certain undesirable foods from your children's diets, you may have better success educating your children about the benefits of eating good food and drinking copious amounts of pure water.

Sometimes parents have to be creative in the dissemination of this type of information. It can often be more effective if children discover these facts on their own, perhaps by reading an article that just happens to be lying open on a coffee table. Soon they will be trying to motivate their parents to drink more water. This is why good parenting often requires extraordinary "SUPER-VISION."

Water Cravings

When children come home from school and forage for a snack, the question parents might ask is, "Are my children really hungry or are they thirsty?" Research has been done to try to tease out the answer to this question. In one study at the University of Washington, subjects who woke up during the night feeling hungry were asked to drink an 8-ounce glass of water and then wait 15 minutes. If they were still hungry, then they were allowed to eat. The majority of the subjects were more often than not completely satisfied by the water and subsequently went back to sleep. This result indicates that our hunger pangs are not always what they appear to be.

The difference between the feelings of hunger and thirst can be difficult to discern. This is partly due to the fact that the satiety or hunger centers in the brain are located right next to the thirst centers. In one report, it was said that 80% of cravings for food are actually cravings for water or feelings of thirst. So when we feel thirsty we are definitely craving the hydrating effect of water, but even when we feel hungry, we may also be craving water more than food.

Another explanation for the blending of the sensations of hunger and thirst is that water is a significant component of the food we eat. Fruits and vegetables contain between 70% and 95% water—even bread is 35% water. When we eat, we take in nutrients and calories, and we obtain water. Therefore, it's possible that when we crave a piece of Italian bread, we may be in fact craving a glass of water.

Water, No Ice, Please!

The great American thirst-quencher is a large glass of ice water, iced tea, or lemonade. The reality is that when it comes to hydrating the body, the colder the beverage is, the less likely it will be able to properly hydrate you. A cold drink may cool you off but it will not rehydrate you if you have just finished exercising or spent time in the hot sun. Cold water constricts the esophagus and stomach, compromising absorption and ultimately hydration. In Ayurveda, it is said that cold water puts out the digestive fire, making it harder to digest your food. This is also true from an enzymatic point of view. Our digestive enzymes function optimally at body temperature; when we cool the digestive system by drinking iced drinks, it interferes with the ability of the enzymes to properly digest our food.

So eating a pizza at eight o'clock at night with a large glass of iced, dehydrating cola is a tall order for a 12-year-old's digestive system. The cold drink will slow the digestive system. When your child wakes up with a stomachache or allergy attack the morning, you'll know why.

Practically speaking, cold water won't really harm your digestive system. But when you layer a heavy meal—eaten late at night with ice cream for dessert—on top of a stressful day, you'll start to see the accumulation of factors that wear on the body and promote disease.

Each person is different, so your role as a parent is to decipher which of these factors will most directly and severely impact your individual child. Cold water may be devastating for one child to drink because of its effects on digestion, while it seems not to affect another child. Knowing your child's kid-type can provide insight into explaining these differences.

> Cold drinks can be a treat during the sunny days of summer. The summer heat provides enough warmth both inside and outside the body so you have the luxury of breaking the cold-drink rule more often; nature provides enough heat to offset any irritating effects from the ice-cold water.

According to Ayurveda, the most effective hydrating beverage is plain hot water. This may not be practical when you need to drink several glasses of water each day, so drink room-temperature water. The next time you are at a restaurant, ask for a glass of water with "no ice" so that before your meal you won't drown your body's digestive ability in a cold bath of ice and soda pop. If you encourage your children to start drinking water without ice when they are young, they will get used to it, and even prefer it. Iced water is an American drink. If you ask for water in a restaurant in Europe, they will bring you a carafe of room-temperature water and glasses without ice.

> When you and your family give it a chance, you will find that room-temperature water is easier to drink and tastes better.

The Effect of Pure Water on Obesity

If a child is dehydrated and the body is searching for water and the satisfaction of hydration, the body will do everything it can to hold onto water. Often in obesity, a large%age of the excess weight is water the body is hoarding. This can be gracefully remedied by making water the primary drink of choice. Soon the body will become rehydrated and the need to hold onto the excess water will be relieved.

I recently worked with a man who weighed 525 pounds and wanted to lose weight. He came to me because he had read my book, *The 3-Season Diet*. I gave him some deceptively simple instructions. I asked him to eat a small breakfast, one that would just be sufficient to see him through to lunchtime without hunger. Then I asked him to eat a significantly larger lunch, one that would make the midday meal the largest and final meal of the day. When he asked me if I was crazy, I assured him I was not. I told him that if he was hungry in the evening it was because he did not have a big enough lunch or he was not drinking enough water.

Two days later he called and said that he was amazed because his nighttime cravings had disappeared.

He noticed that if he were just a little bit hungry, all he would need to do is drink a large glass of water and his hunger pangs would pass. In a year and a half he dropped from 525 to 350 pounds. He said he never felt hungry or deprived—he realized how important his water intake was. If he felt hungry, the only thing that would alleviate the hunger pangs was pure water; not even natural juice would do the trick. The state of chronic dehydration his body had experienced previously caused it to compensate with excessive weight gain and fluid retention.

Obesity and the associated risk

> A very simple weight-loss and junkfood avoidance technique for kids is to drink a glass of water when they are hungry for a snack and then wait 10 or 15 minutes. If they are still hungry, then feed them. More often than not, within ten minutes, they'll be off playing as if the hunger pangs never existed.

factors for diabetes are becoming epidemic in our American culture. Children as young as 10 years old are regularly being diagnosed with type II, or adult-onset diabetes, a disease once reserved for overweight and sedentary older adults. Now obese and overweight children are commonly diagnosed with this form of diabetes caused by improper diet and lifestyle. While obesity rates have doubled in the United States in the last twenty years the number of people with type II diabetes has increased by one-third in the 1990s.

The Magic of Water

Let's look at some of the essential functions of water in the human body:

- Maintains the structure and function of DNA
- Allows for oxygen to be delivered to the cell
- Is essential for the manufacture of proteins involved in tissue growth and repair
- Enables repair proteins to rebuild the cellular structure
- Acts as a medium for the transport of nutrients
- Cushions bones and joints
- Lubricates joints
- Provides a medium for the removal of waste products
- Allows for the maintenance of the cells' normal electrical conductivity
- Regulates body temperature
- Hydrates the cells
- Supports the immune system
- Allows for proper maintenance of the basal metabolic rate
- Acts as a medium for the body to eliminate free radicals
- Is an important ingredient in digestive juices

When adequate amounts of water are available in the body, equal osmotic pressure is created and maintained between the water-based intra-cellular and extra-cellular fluids. But when the body is dehydrated, the sodium-rich extra-cellular fluids leach water from the cells. This causes the depletion of the water from the potassium-rich intra-cellular fluid, compromising energy production and cellular function. As fluid is leached out of the cells, it causes swelling, edema, and water retention.

The Hydration Equation

How Can You Tell If Your Children Are Properly Hydrated?

If children are properly hydrated, they will urinate at least six times a day. The color of urine should be clear, or a very pale yellow. If it is dark-colored and less frequent, the child may be dehydrated.

If your children feel thirsty, their bodies are already in the early stages of dehydration. And as the body becomes more dehydrated, thirst becomes an increasingly unreliable indicator of your children's water needs.

If you wait to give your children water until they are thirsty, you have waited too long to give them water. In the same way we need to treat a cold while the child is still healthy, we need to treat dehydration when the body is still hydrated.

Athletes have a particularly difficult time knowing how much water to drink in order to be properly hydrated for a particular event, and thirst is a particularly unreliable reflection of the body's water needs during training or athletic events. The result has been millions of dollars spent on the development of sports drinks.

How Much Water To Drink?

According to research done at Cornell University Medical Center for Nutritional Information, Americans, on average, consume 7.9 servings of hydrating beverages and 4.9 servings of dehydrating beverages each day.

The average daily consumption of hydrating beverages are:

- Water   4.6 servings
- Milk   1.3 servings
- Carbonated soda without caffeine   0.6 servings
- Juices   1.4 servings
- TOTAL   **7.9 servings**

The average daily consumption of dehydrating beverages are:

• Coffee	1.8 servings
• Tea	1.0 servings
• Carbonated soda with caffeine	1.3 servings
• Beer	0.5 servings
• Wine or other alcoholic beverages	0.3 servings
• **TOTAL**	**4.9 servings**

Statistically, the average American is drinking only three servings of hydrating beverages a day—which is simply not enough to hydrate a body made up of 78% water. According to Steven Meyerowitz, author of *Water, the Ultimate Cure,* the water content of the body is as follows: the adult body contains 40 to 50 quarts of water. The blood is 83% water, muscles 75%, brain 75%, heart 75%, bones 22%, lungs 86%, kidneys 83%, and eyes 95%.

Maintaining the levels of water in our body is something that takes daily intake of water. We lose between 2 and 3 quarts of water a day just through non-exertion perspiration and evaporation. If we exercise or exert ourselves, we can lose twice that amount. Water loss during exercise can be deceiving. We sweat even when it is cold outside, and this water loss can have immediate effects on the body. One study performed with athletes showed that if they lost 2% of their body weight through water loss during exercise, they would experience a 25% decrease in strength and athletic performance.

For kids who exercise, a good rule of thumb is to drink 16 ounces of water for every pound lost while exercising. To measure this, use the scale found in most clubs or school gyms to complete a pre- and post-workout "weigh-in." After a few weigh-ins, you or your child will be able to judge fairly accurately how much water is needed to replenish the water lost during exercise.

When my 15-year-old daughter, a basketball player, learned that there is a 25% decrease in athletic performance for every 2% loss in body weight due to perspiration, she began filling two 32-ounce water bottles to take to school.

> To stay properly hydrated and avoid dehydration: divide your body weight in pounds by two. This gives the number of ounces of pure water you should drink each day to stay hydrated. This is in addition to other fluids, fruits, or juices you drink during the day. For example, if you weigh 120 pounds, you need to drink 60 ounces (about 2 quarts) of pure water daily.

Chronic Dehydration

It is critically important for the health of everybody, adults and children alike, to stay fully hydrated. If the body is not fully hydrated, there are a number of different signs and symptoms both of the early and chronic stages of dehydration that will appear. The following lists comes from Steve Meyerowitz's book, *Water*.

Symptoms of dehydration:

- Fatigue
- Anxiety
- Irritability
- Depression
- Cravings
- Muscle cramps
- Headaches

Mature or chronic symptoms of dehydration:

- Heartburn
- Joint and back pain
- Migraine headaches
- Fibromyalgia
- Constipation
- Colitis

Signs of chronic emergency dehydration:

- Asthma
- Allergies
- Diabetes

- Autoimmune diseases
- Psoriasis
- Lupus
- Eczema

Note: Acute dehydration is an actual medical emergency, as we will die—in about three days—from lack of water. During hot days, high altitudes, or conditions of exertion, even low levels of acute dehydration can contribute to medical emergencies like heat exhaustion or heat stroke. The above lists are the stages, symptoms, and conditions linked to chronic and degenerative dehydration.

Asthma and Allergies

Chronic dehydration can worsen conditions that can result in chronic asthma or allergies or an acute asthma attack. There are a few interconnected mechanisms by which dehydration can lead to the development of, or exacerbate, existing allergies and asthma. We are familiar with the body systems involved: the lymphatic and immune systems, as well as the mucous membranes of the respiratory tract. Let's examine these as they are related to dehydration.

We know that the mucous membranes need to be constantly moist, but if the body is dehydrated, they are unable to remain moist and well lubricated. This dryness caused by dehydration triggers the body's histamine response leading to the production of excessive mucus in the sinuses and digestive tract as well as edema and swelling in body, particularly in the small air sacs (alveoli) of the lungs. The swelling and edema leads to the constriction of airflow in the bronchioles, causing shortness of breath. Labored breathing or wheezing is the first sign of an asthmatic attack.

Asthma can be dramatically affected through hydration, as shown by the following case study cited by Julian Whitaker, M.D., in the *Health & Healing Newsletter*: "After only four days of drinking eight glasses of water each day, 8-year-old Jeremy's asthma cleared up to the extent that he was able to discontinue all of his medications. Within one month his lung capacity increased from

60% of normal to 120% ... Arthritis, ulcers, edema, and even blood pressure—I have seen them all improve with water."

Dehydration also interferes with the ability of the lymphatic system to drain properly. If the lymphatic system, which both removes wastes and hosts the immune system, is not functioning properly, the body becomes hypersensitive to potential irritants like pollens, pollutants, and allergens. Just as the dryness in the mucous membranes triggers a histamine response, the sluggish lymphatic fluid and build-up of irritants triggers a histamine response.

The histamine response is the body's classic allergic response, causing the production of even more mucus and fluids to protect the cells from a potential threat. The key to resolving a chronic allergy is not allowing the body produce the histamine in the first place. Although this may seem like an impossible task, what it requires is an efficient waste-removal and a lymphatic system that effectively drains the tissues and promotes a powerful immune system. Proper hydration is the first and most fundamental step in keeping the lymphatic system moving and preventing the cells from developing hypersensitivities.

Allergic problems include skin toxicity. Many children experience hives when they are having an allergic reaction because of the connection between waste removal and the lymphatic drainage of the skin (discussed in Chapters 3 and 4). When this drainage is compromised, the skin can become a toxic-release valve, causing hives, eczema, and rashes in children. In adults, the lymphatic fluid commonly stores these impurities in the muscles, creating stiffness, fatigue, and, if chronic, fibromyalgia. A sluggish lymphatic system can be directly traced to a chronic state of dehydration. This can be exacerbated in children who are sedentary, which we will review in Chapter 11 when I discuss play.

The high water content of the supple, water balloon-like body of fully hydrated babies is not the only explanation for their flexibility and softness. Their well-hydrated lymphatic systems effectively move toxins through their bodies. When the body is dehydrated and the lymphatic system is sluggish, toxins that are unable to be released get stored in the body, especially in the muscles. Soon the muscles become dehydrated and stiff, and slowly lose their blood supply. Without an adequate blood supply, the muscles lay down scar tissue and lose their elasticity, dramatically increasing the amount of effort needed to contract the muscle. The body loses strength and energy and its susceptibility to allergic conditions and chronic illness increases.

Hydration and Digestion

In the last chapter I talked about the importance of having a balanced digestive system. Proper hydration is an essential part of having a balanced and healthy digestive system. Our stomach is an amazing and durable organ, miraculously able to digest the things we put into our mouths. The stomach contains incredibly powerful acids to be able to accomplish this. The acidity of the stomach is crucial for digestion as the acids complete the first step in the breakdown of food, especially heavy foods like proteins and fats. It also kills many harmful bacteria and other microorganisms.

The stomach has a thick mucus layer that protects the lining against these powerful acids. Beneath the mucus are glandular cells that produce a bicarbonate solution that deposits into the mucus layer, protecting the stomach's lining from acids. If a child is dehydrated, the stomach mucus and bicarbonate solution can become deficient, triggering a histamine response of excess mucus and stomach backpressure. This is one dehydration-based cause of stomachaches.

> The stomach acids are so strong that if the mucusy and alkaline buffer layer protecting the stomach fails, the acids quickly burn a hole right through the stomach wall.

 Remember: Your children should be drinking one-half their body weight in ounces of water each day. This is above and beyond any juices and soda pops they drink.

If acids were allowed to leave to the stomach and move into an unprepared small intestine, they would do irreparable damage to the intestinal wall. The small intestine does not have the same thick acid-protecting layer of mucus as the stomach. To protect itself, the small intestine contains an alkaline environment designed to neutralize stomach acids. This environment is maintained by the watery bicarbonate solution produced and released by the pancreas. The pancreas ensures that the small intestine is sufficiently alkaline before the pyloric sphincter, which separates the small intestine from the stomach, opens. Ample amounts of water are needed to manufacture and maintain this bicarbonate solution.

If a child is dehydrated, it becomes more difficult for the pancreas to manufacture these fluids. When the stomach fills with food, and the acids build up after a child eats a large meal of pizza and ice cream, if the small intestine is not ready to neutralize these acids the pyloric sphincter tightens and food gets backed up in the stomach. When this happens, the child says, "I have a tummyache!"

If this food pressure in the stomach is not released, the child commonly begins to feel nauseous as the pyloric sphincter tightens and the food that is trying to leave the stomach is forced to stay. The body is serious about not letting the acidic stomach contents leave until the small intestine is adequately prepared to receive them. This often occurs when the small intestine has not produced the proper alkaline environment necessary to neutralize these stomach acids. More often than not, this is related to low water consumption and dehydration.

When the body will not allow food to move into the small intestine, the ring valve between the stomach and esophagus relaxes in order to release pressure in the stomach by letting some of the food back up into the esophagus. At this point, food is not the only thing filling the stomach; the buildup of stomach acids triggers multiple histamine receptors in

> At this point the best medicine parents can give their children is a large glass of water. After 10 to 15 minutes, give them another glass.

the stomach lining, stimulating the production of an increased amount of protective mucus, and even further increasing the pressure that is building up in the stomach. This is when your child says, "I think I'm going to throw up."

At this point it may be too late for your child to drink a glass of water. It might be the best thing for the child to throw up and reset the digestive process. Throwing up is a natural cleansing action triggered by the body. It can be caused by dehydration, overeating, a stomach virus, or what is commonly called food poisoning, which is the presence of some kind of contaminant in the food.

A Word on Constipation

In the digestive system, one of the primary roles of the small intestine is to absorb nutrients from our food into the bloodstream. Many essential nutrients are water-soluble, and a watery medium is required for their absorption. The lining of the intestinal tract must perform the delicately balanced task of absorbing these nutrients out of the watery solution. The large intestine further completes the process of digestion by absorbing specific nutrients and any remaining water, leaving the residual waste neither too dry nor too loose, but properly balanced for elimination.

Dehydration triggers a series of hormonal reactions, telling the body to hold on to as much water as possible. Water is retained, the body swells, mucus-producing histamines are released, and the intestines, masters of pulling water out of food, sometimes overdo it. Soon both the intestinal wall and the stools become overly dried out, leading to constipation. Water is a well-known remedy for constipation, used by alternative and modern medicine alike as the first treatment against chronic constipation for both children and adults.

> It is important for a parent to understand the role water plays in keeping a child's digestive system balanced. Stomachaches and nausea are often easily prevented simply by keeping your child properly hydrated.

Different Types of Available Water

Mineral Water—water that has large quantities of minerals, naturally collected by passing through various layers of earth and rocks to a well or spring. According to the FDA, to be labeled as such, mineral water must have at least 250 ppm (parts per million) total dissolved solids (minerals dissolved into the water as a solution). Water with a high mineral content often has a stronger taste. There are debates over how much mineral content makes this water most beneficial for the human body. Too many minerals may be deposited in the deep tissues and not absorbed into the cells, but absorbing minerals into the body is a difficult task. What better way to make minerals available on a cellular level then to dissolve them in water? This debate is ongoing.

Spring Water—water that flows naturally from an underground spring without the use of drilling or wells. Each spring water company has its own theory about why its water is better than others. The amount of dissolved minerals in these waters differs greatly. By federal regulation, every bottled spring water, mineral water, or filtered water must be treated for bacteria before it can be bottled or sold.

If you want to drink bottled water that is untouched by humans without any treatments for bacteria or filtration, Trinity is the only one that I am aware of currently on the market. Trinity is the brand name of bottled water that is so pure that the founder, Jock Bell, was not willing to subject his water to bactericidal treatments, which he would have to do if it were labeled as spring water. He claimed that his water was a dietary supplement and therefore did not need to be treated or irradiated for bacteria, and he successfully lobbied the FDA to create a new classification of bottled water. So if you are looking for water in its most natural untouched state, look for a local spring or buy pure bottled water that has not been altered.

Filtered Water—this water is usually from a municipal water source, but it has been filtered and treated using a variety of different purification and filtration systems.

Municipal Water—water supplied by a city for public use, stored in a reservoir, and then delivered to home taps and faucets. Unfortunately, most municipal water supplies are treated with chlorine, disinfectants, and often fluoride. The effectiveness, health benefits, and risks of these types of treatment are controversial and are being debated.

Water Treatment

There are several techniques to remove bacteria, microorganisms, and chemicals from water. Here are a few of the most common techniques used by municipalities, bottled water companies, and home filtration systems.

Carbon Filtration (same as a charcoal filter)—Carbon ash is condensed and the water is filtered through it. This process removes pollutants and pesticides and is beneficial for removing toxic odors and undesirable tastes. Some carbon-block filters (especially those with sub-micron strainers) can remove bacteria and heavy metals such as lead, cadmium, and chromium. Since this process relies on a filter, it is important to change the filter frequently as it can be a potential breeding ground for bacteria (although it may be difficult to know when a new filter is needed). It is also important to take care of the filter; which may break down with extended use or by hot water running through it. One of the drawbacks of carbon filtration is that it cannot remove fluorides. So if you are drinking fluoridated water and want to remove the fluoride, you need to use an alternative filtration system such as distillation.

Ultraviolet Light—one of the most commonly used water treatments for bottled water. UV light is lethal to bacteria, viruses, and other microbial organisms. It is a quick and inexpensive way of ensuring that the public will not be unintentionally exposed to pathogens. UV lights are installed in bottling plants, and before the water enters the bottle, it is irradiated by the ultraviolet light. The downside of UV light purification is that if the water is really pure, the UV light will neutralize the trace element vibrational qualities that can make the water unique.

Ozone (O₃)—an unstable molecule formed when oxygen (O_2) is agitated and split. Ozone is considered to be one of the most powerful bactericidal agents. It also oxidizes pesticides and chlorine, removing them from the water while precipitating out heavy metals and fluorides.

Chlorine—one of the most common, if not *the* most common, water purification techniques. Chlorine is an effective treatment for bacteria but not as useful for larger organisms like cysts, amoebae, and protozoa. According to medical dictionaries, chlorine is a disinfectant, deodorant, and irritant poison. It is a good idea not to drink chlorinated water, so if your municipal water system uses chlorination, try an inexpensive filtration system.

Distilled Water—water that has been purified by being passed through an evaporative-condensation cycle. Home distillers can be purchased that remove all bacteria and microorganisms including viruses, fluorides, heavy metals, and pesticides. Basically, distilled water removes everything. The problem is that once the water is purified, even contact with the currently polluted atmosphere will contaminate it. This can happen easily because pure water is a sticky molecule that constantly attracts hitchhikers. Hundreds of years ago before the environment became so polluted, naturally distilled rainwater was probably one of the safest and best drinking waters. Currently, there is a debate over whether it is safe to drink distilled water for extended periods of time. Some people claim that distilled water will slowly leach minerals out of the body, leaving it depleted. There seems to be compelling research on both sides of this debate.

Structured Water—new high-tech bottled water that claims to organize water molecules into crystalline structures mimicking water found in the cytoplasm of healthy cells and in healing sources of water around the world. These waters are typically very expensive, and although they may have great benefits, they are generally unproven and out of the price range for most families to drink on a regular basis.

Water filtration is a very complicated and confusing subject, especially since each water bottler and purification system claims to have the best water treatment system. It is not within the scope of this book to go into detail about each treatment system available. There are other books that are excellent resources and offer more information on this subject. Two books that I recommend are: *Water, the Ultimate Cure* by Steve Meyerowitz, and *Your Water and Your Health* by Allen Bank.

An Ancient Water Treatment

A simple way to ensure that you are drinking pure and safe water is to use of an inexpensive carbon filter and boil your water. The filter can be a small sink unit or one that fits on top of a pitcher of water and filters as you drink. To finish the job of purifying your water, boil it for 10 to 15 minutes. The technique of boiling water in preparation for drinking has been used since ancient times, even when water sources were much more pure than they are now.

Today we realize that the technique of boiling water kills bacteria and other microorganisms and boils off carcinogens. Traditionally, water was free of cancer-causing substances, and in most cases a bacteria-free water source was used. Yet, it was still customary to boil water prior to drinking. Ayurvedic thought is that boiling makes the water lighter and more refined in some way. It was understood that boiling water would allow it to be more effectively assimilated and used by the body. Clearly, this technique will boil off undesirable passengers that have hooked on the water molecule. The process of boiling water removes excess chemicals, bacteria, heavy metals, and minerals.

Removing hitchhikers from water molecules relates to the recently identified aquaporins, or small pores in the cell membrane, which were mentioned at the beginning of the chapter. These aquaporins are ports of hydration for the cell and are exclusive channels for pure water—composed only of one oxygen and two hydrogen atoms. Before any water is able to enter the aquaporins of the cell membrane, it must be stripped of its unnecessary and often toxic baggage.

Remember: Dehydration is a major cause of chronic and recurrent health conditions.

To prevent dehydration (for parents and children alike):

- Don't wait until feeling thirsty to drink—by this time the body is already two to three cups of water low.
- Start and end each day with one full glass of water. This is important because the body loses water during the night.
- Send kids to school with a bottle of water rather than juice.
- Do your best to drink a glass of water one-half hour or so before each meal.
- Drink a glass of water two hours after eating a meal.
- Sip water during meals.
- Avoid caffeinated beverages, which dehydrate the body.
- Increase water consumption in hot weather and during and after exercise.
- Drink half your body weight in ounces each day.
- Always drink the purest water available.
- Drink more while sick or under stress.
- When drinking juice, it is best to drink freshly squeezed or freshly juiced fruits and vegetables—but they do not replace water.
- Drink room-temperature water—not iced water or drinks.

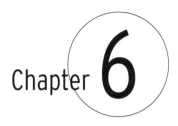

Chapter 6

Secret 5—Moods and Weight Balancing

Have your kids ever come home from school famished and started scrounging around for something—anything—to eat? Once they have a snack, do you have a hard time getting them to focus on their homework? Are they seldom hungry for dinner? Do they resist going to bed because they aren't sleepy? Are they difficult to get up in the morning?

Each day our bodies ride a rapidly flowing river of changing hormone levels. These hormone levels fluctuate from the time we get up in the morning to the time we go to bed, and continue to fluctuate throughout the night. These are the body's circadian rhythms. This chapter describes the fifth health secret—how to go with the flow of our bodies' natural cycles.

We will see in this chapter that there are some times that are better than others for eating, exercising, going to bed, and doing homework, based on the rhythms of the day. Some simple modifications in the structure of your children's lives can go a long way toward taking the pandemonium out of your home life.

When our children seem to be hungry or tired at the wrong times, or full of spit and vinegar when they should be doing homework, it may simple be a matter of resetting their routine. Instead of paddling the boat upstream against the current of the body's natural rhythms, children can learn to row gently downstream.

To set ourselves smoothly on the river, it is important to understand our connection to the rhythms and cycles of nature. This connection, through the ebb and flow of our hormones during the course of the day and from season to season, once dictated very smoothly and spontaneously the daily and seasonal routines that sustained human life for many thousands of years.

It is only recently, in the last 30 to 40 years, that we have almost completely forgotten the laws of the land. People experience life as a struggle when they choose to swim against the current of these natural cycles. In this chapter, I will show you how to carry on a standard child-rearing routine while maintaining respect for the cycles of nature.

> Jet lag is just one example of moving against the natural cycle. The discomfort and disorientation is merely the experience of a body tuned into one set of rhythms that in a few short hours is plunked down in the middle of a new set of natural rhythms. It takes the body a few days to reset the hormonal cycles and be in rhythm with the new sunrise and sunset.

Mom! I'm Home!

When kids come home from school after a long day of stress, classes, homework, tests, and play, the very first thing they do is to go straight to the refrigerator or snack cupboard to seek out and consume their snack of choice. If there is nothing wholesome prepared and available, then the snack is often something like cookies and milk, or a piece of cake. The worst time to go to the grocery store is when you're hungry, because you fill your cart with sugar-laced comfort foods you would typically refrain from buying. Likewise, when hungry kids come home from school, they will eat the first thing they find.

If we do not have something healthful prepared and ready for them, their low blood sugar will entice their minds to find instant gratification with energy-filled, sugar-laced snacks—even if those snacks are hidden from view. Within a few short minutes after eating, their blood sugar level begins to rise. Most sugar-based comfort foods overshoot the mark. Instead of just satisfying the cravings, the blood sugar injection over-stimulates the child's nervous system. This over-stimulation leads to mayhem. Suddenly siblings can't seem to get along. When you ask your kids to do their homework, they may go to their rooms and open their books, but they will be easily distracted. If your lucky, the weather will be nice and you can send them outside to burn off some of their steam. Exercising when the blood sugar levels are high is your child's best medicine to calm down. Unfortunately, most kids find their simulative outlets through video games or zoning out in front of the TV.

By dinnertime at six o'clock, the blood sugar level has now sunk to a new low. When children sit down for dinner in the midst of a sugar craving, vegetables are the enemy. You become frustrated with your attempts to force-feed your kids green beans, salad, rice, and fried chicken. Dinnertime, instead of being a peaceful experience of eating and sharing, becomes a disciplinary venue as you try to convince your kids that they have to eat all the food on their plate.

If this sounds even remotely familiar, you may want to find a better way to motivate your children to eat, sleep, and do homework without all the fuss. Let's face it, as parents we do the best we can to feed our kids a healthy breakfast and pack them a good lunch or give them lunch money so they can buy a hot lunch at school. This works in theory; but in practice, the amount of their lunch that actually gets ingested is one of those unsolved mysteries. We encourage them to eat their entire lunch, but we are left with no guarantees. More often than not, lunch boxes come home only half-eaten at best.

With five school-age children in our family, it has become extremely clear to me that what happens at lunchtime is uncontrollable and unpredictable. As parents, we come to realize that if we rely on a school lunch to provide proper nutrition for our children, we are making a large dietary mistake. For most children, lunch is a random experience. In many cases, kids only have 10 to 15 minutes to eat their meal before they must clear out of the cafeteria. With the social pressure of: "Who am I going to sit next to?" and "Will I fit in and be included today on the playground?" lunch is not always the best time to digest a meal, at least from an emotional perspective. Our bodies prefer to sit down and eat a meal in a relaxed, non-distracting and non-threatening environment. A lunch room typically provides the least relaxed and most distracting environment your child will experience all day. Yet, we expect our children to be able to block out all of these distractions, sit down in a relaxed way, and enjoy the lunch we prepared for them with such love and devotion.

If there is one thing you can count on with regard to your kids' hunger, it is that they will eat just about anything when they come home from school. In our house, we find that if we feed the kids at this time of day, between three and four o'clock,they will eat everything we give them, even the green stuff. Not only in Ayurveda, but throughout the world for thousands of years, lunch was (and in many places still is) the main meal of the day. Even in America, up until our relatively recent shift from an agricultural to an industrial culture, we ate our largest meal of the day during at midday.

Most of us find ourselves paddling upstream all day long. Life is a struggle for many of us, and.our children learn significantly through our example. If they see us coming home from work exhausted and feeling high levels of stress, then this is the mental mindset that is being conditioned in their brains.

To change the day's routine from an endless struggle to a smooth series of transitions, we need to understand the natural flow of the daily cycle.

In Chapter 7, I will discuss the seasonal rhythms of nature that support all life on earth. We are connected to these natural cycles just as the birds are connected to their migration cycles. Their lives depend on their instinctual adher-

ence to these cycles. What if the
birds decided not to fly south
for the winter? Birds don't
debate their migration patterns,
or at which island in the
Bahamas they will winter.
Without a built-in mechanism
to follow the seasonal rhythms,
birds and other species that
depend on migration would slowly die off.

> Fortunately, when you live life in harmony, sailing downstream with the flow of these natural cycles, you do not have to wait years to feel the difference; you'll notice the change instantly in your own lives and the lives of your children.

Humans are no strangers to adhering to nature's cycles.
Throughout history, traditional people, even many American farmers, lived naturally and effortlessly in harmony with the cycles.
Foods were eaten in season and the diet changed for each season.
People slept and woke with the sun. The Native American
Cherokees went to bed two hours after sunset, meaning that they
slept more in the winter, which prepared them for the activity of
spring and summer. In the summer, when days were long and nights
were short, they slept less, drawing on their reserves that were
stored in their bodies during the winter months.

These very powerful cycles still exist, and the lives and survival
of traditional people still depend on living harmoniously with them.
In our modern world, we have, with great efficiency, insulated ourselves from these natural cycles without really realizing it. But living
life against the current of these cycles over many years slowly
takes its toll, creating strain, struggle, and imbalance. This happens
so gradually that we don't recognize the cause of this strain.

Secret 5: The fifth health secret is to integrate our routines with the
ebb and flow of our hormonal cycles as mandated by the daily cycles
of nature. People experience life as a struggle because they choose to
swim against the current of life's natural cycles. By living life in harmony and flowing downstream with nature's rhythms, you can eliminate significant amounts of stress from our children's lives.

Just as the qualities of winter, spring, and summer cycle through our lives (described in Chapter 3), these qualities also cycle throughout the day. In order to have a daily routine that runs smoothly—free from mayhem, cravings, and blood sugar fluctuations—and incorporates stamina, sound sleep, and a clear head, it is important to understand the daily cycles.

The Daily Cycles

Let's start and finish with the sunrise and sunset. Even though, in the U.S., the times of sunrise and sunset fluctuate throughout the year, we will define the segments of the day by calling 6 A.M. sunrise and 6 P.M. sunset. (In Chapter 7 we will discuss the implications of the shorter winter and longer summer days.)

6 A.M.–10 A.M.	SPRING—KAPHA
10 A.M.–2 P.M.	SUMMER—PITTA
2 P.M.–6 P.M.	WINTER—VATA
6 P.M.–10 P.M.	SPRING—KAPHA
10 P.M.–2 A.M.	SUMMER—PITTA
2 A.M.–6 A.M.	WINTER—VATA

The Human Punch Clock

We begin the day with sunrise. Just as spring is the start of nature's new year, the morning is the springtime of the day. The same properties that support the start of nature's new year support the start of each day. The rains of spring create a moist, humid environment, which allows the rapid growth of a seed as it germinates into a plant. Likewise the body creates more mucus in the morning to lubricate the body, including runny noses for some people upon waking up. Our bodies are naturally stronger (but stiff) in the morning, making exercise—including some gentle stretching—a great way to start the day. This morning spring cycle lasts from about 6 A.M. to 10 A.M.

The next cycle is the midday summer cycle from 10 A.M. to 2 P.M. This is the time of the day when the sun is highest in the sky and the fiery digestive system is at its most efficient and powerful. This is the time of day when it is easiest for us to digest a large meal to provide fuel for the rest of the day.

The winter cycle, from 2 P.M. until 6 P.M., completes the first half of the 24-hour daily cycle, starting at sunrise and ending with sunset. These afternoon winter hours are associated with the busy, energy-hungry nervous system, which is why we may feel a lull if we are not properly fortified with fuel.

The three cycles repeat themselves in the second half of the daily cycle, from sunset to sunrise. From 6 P.M. to 10 P.M., the heavy spring qualities increase, slowing the metabolism and prepare the body for sleep. From 10 P.M. until 2 A.M.,the hot summer cycle is activated, often triggering midnight snacking and the energy that fuels night owls. The midnight summer cycle is actually a time when the body initiates a cleansing process. The liver releases enzymes, such as glutathione peroxidase, that detoxify the day's accumulated impurities in the body. These enzymes are the body's night janitor, who cleans floors and washes windows in order to prepare for the following day.

The final cycle, from 2 A.M. until 6 A.M., culminates with the sunrise and is a time when the winter nervous system cycle repeats itself. The nervous system uses this time to begin waking the body. This is also the portion of the night when our active mind spends the most time in dream-rich REM (Rapid Eye Movement) sleep. Many people take advantage of the early morning mental alertness by getting up and engaging in creative thought or meditation and prayer.

Rise and Shine

A parent's life would be so much easier if kids went to bed on time and got out of bed in the morning after only one request to wake up. But kids often stay up late and can't seem to get up in the morning, lingering in bed long after sunrise. There is a reason why children can't seem to muster themselves out from under the sheets: the longer you sleep after sunrise the sleepier, heavier, and more sluggish you feel.

After sunrise, the spring cycle of the morning begins. Remember that your children are in the spring cycle of their lives, so trying to get out of bed has the combined effects of all the heavy spring qualities, making it more difficult for them than for adults. Adults have grown out of the spring lifecycle and will find it easier to wake up and function even if they sleep past sunrise into the spring cycle morning hours. I should mention that these are the general tendencies, and the influence of different body types and individual situations may cause these tendencies not to be as clearly expressed as they are written, but the general tendencies are there.

Your child's kid-type will also play a major role in their willingness to get out of bed in the morning. A parent's biggest challenge will be waking a spring kid-type in the midst of the spring lifecycle during one of the spring months of the year. To remedy this situation, the child must go to bed early, so you can wake him or her as early as possible. If this child is allowed to sleep in, he or she will be more difficult to wake.

Staying in bed too long in the morning also increases inflexibility in the body. The mucus-intensive spring hours of the morning support the qualities of heaviness and solidity in the body that serve as shock absorbers so people can withstand the physical labor of plowing fields, digging ditches, and physical exercise. The longer someone lies in bed in the morning, the stiffer these "shock absorbers" become, and as a result, the more stiff and lethargic the person can become. Getting up early avoids the influence of the heavy spring morning cycle on the body's flexibility.

If we started our day before or right around sunrise, we would be up-and-at-'em before the heavy spring cycle kicked in with its stiffness, lethargy, and increased sleepiness. I am sure everyone has experienced a time in their lives when they woke up early, before sunrise, and felt great: light, flexible, and full of energy.

 Remember the old saying: "Early to bed, early to rise, makes you healthy, wealthy, and wise."

In most cultures, being awake to watch the day start (around sunrise) is a regular practice. Only Westernized cultures advocate sleeping in past sunrise on a regular basis. The key to rising earlier is to get the kids to bed early. A great example of this is when you go camping. All of a sudden, even the sworn "night people" are in bed early and up in the morning with the sun. Once you remove all the modern distractions of lights, TV, and stereos, early to bed and early to rise is a natural state of being.

> I am not saying that that your children must be up before sunrise. However, cultivating the habit of going to bed early and naturally waking up early is a routine to strive for.

Starting the Day

Waking up as early as possible and engaging in some physical activity in the morning provides a baseline of stability and balance for the body's hormones, blood sugar levels, and fat-burning metabolism. When the sun rises, the body's hormones start to prepare for the day and gear up the body for physical activity. Studies in the Soviet Union have shown that the muscles are in fact stronger during the morning hours between 6 A.M. and 10 A.M. Many people might say just the opposite because their experience in the morning is one of being tired and dragging, not full of muscular strength; but this morning cycle is nature's way of facilitating physical activity.

For people who work on farms, a day that starts after the sunrise is unheard of. The majority of the physical labor on farms is done in the morning and evening to avoid the strong midday heat. The morning hours are the physical hours. We have an easier time sustaining a routine of physical activity in the morning than any other time of the day. In fact, one study showed that 75% of people in America who had a regular morning exercise routine were still exercising one year later. Only 25% of the people who exercised at other times of the day had a regular exercise routine one year later.

The fuel that the body uses most effectively for physical exercise is fat—not sugar. If a child were to start the day with even 5 or 10 minutes of proper physical activity, it would cause the body to shift into a fat-burning metabolism. Participating in P.E. class in the morning helps support a mood-stabilizing, fat-burning metabolism. If a child begins the day without exercise but with sugar-filled cereals, the results will be reversed. Sugar-laced comfort foods excessively stimulate the nervous system, setting up the child for blood sugar fluctuations, mood-elevating highs, and energy-sapping lows that compromise focus, self-esteem, and enthusiasm.

A few years ago, I introduced some of these principles to an elementary school. We offered an optional morning P.E. class that started one hour before the regular school start time. The kids who came to this class would not have to attend their regularly scheduled P.E. class later in the day. The first day two kids showed up. The next day four appeared; and the next day, six students came in for the early class. By the week's end we had a dozen kids and almost overnight it seemed that every kid was asking a parent for a ride to school early for this morning P.E. class. It soon became the craze— a large majority of the kids at the school were attending the optional early morning P.E. class. It was a great example of putting the kids in a boat and letting them naturally float downstream with the current, showing how kids, when given a choice in the matter, are naturally attracted to floating downstream. As parents, it is our job to raise our kids in such a way that they naturally adhere to the flow of nature's cycles.

To help children control their weight, it is important to be aware of all of the fat-burning opportunities children experience each day, like the stabilizing effect of early morning exercise provided by the P.E. class. With 22% of American children considered to be obese according to the U.S. Centers for Disease Control and Prevention, and with 65% of American adults being either obese or overweight, it may be beneficial for parents and children alike to start their day with a brief session of exercise. In merely 5 or 10 minutes the body naturally shifts into a fat-burning metabolic state. With a little exercise under your belt, even an imperfect breakfast will deliver a stable source of energy because of the supportive baseline of fat metabolism provided by exercise. This enhances steady energy, the ability to focus, and an even demeanor.

It's Dinner Time!!

Ten-year-old Jason went to a public middle school where hot lunches were served every day. Instead of making Jason a cold sack-lunch, his mother opted to spend the extra money to ensure her son had a healthy meal. One day Jason came home and said to his mom, "Why do I have to eat a hot lunch at lunchtime? Lunchtime is supposed to be a sandwich, not this huge hot thing." Jason continued, "No one else eats a hot meal, why should I?"

Jason's mother told me this story during a consultation. She did not know how to respond to his complaint. I told her that hot lunches exist in schools today because parents were initially reluctant to send their children off to school when they were desperately needed on the farm or ranch to make ends meet. When push came to shove and parents realized the importance of an education, they insisted that the child eat a well-cooked hot meal, just like they would get at home. So the deal was, if their children were going to spend the entire day at school, they had better be fed properly. This tradition lives on in lunch programs, though few people understand or appreciate the logic behind the large midday meal tradition.

Unfortunately, America is one of the few countries that has completely abandoned the traditional eating style of the large midday meal. In the industrialized societies of modern Europe, the day is scheduled around the midday meal. Parents and children go to school at seven or eight o'clock in the morning, then school is out at two o'clock in the afternoon and parents come home from work to be with their children for the largest and most important meal of the day. Typically, one of the parents will go back to work from four o'clock until seven or eight o'clock, at which time they sit down again for the light

> The word "supper" comes from soup, indicating that the evening meal would be a "supplemental" soup-like meal, not a large steak dinner with all the trimmings.

evening meal called supper. In many parts of Europe, a shorter work day is also standard, allowing for an adequate lunch break to eat a substantial midday meal.

There is a tradition in England of afternoon tea at around four o'clock. After the afternoon tea, they have another tea around six or seven o'clock when the kids ask, "What's for tea?" The English actually call their evening supper meal "tea" because it is a small supplemental meal consisting of a cup of tea and something light, like soup, a baked potato, biscuits, half a sandwich, or a snack. Many offices close for an hour to allow people to take their lunch break (which is often called dinner) in the middle of the day to eat a substantial meal. Restaurants have special two- or three-course lunches, and one of the most traditional English meals, the Sunday roast, is a large midday meal. This is quite different compared to the American evening meal, which is the largest of the day.

In Ayurveda, it is customary to eat the largest meal of the day at midday because the digestive system is believed to be most efficient in the summer cycle of the day when the sun is in the middle of the sky. Hormone levels indicate that the metabolism is high and able to digest and assimilate a large amount of food at this time. This is when the body is most successfully nourished, an optimal time to provide it with a good supply of energy and nutrition. Interestingly, one study indicated that the taste buds tasted food most effectively during the midday hours, indicating again that this is the most appropriate time to digest a large meal.

Coffee

After this long lunch, it is traditional to stop and take time to digest the food. In Europe, coffee in the form of espresso is one of the favorite traditional digestives given to help process the large lunchtime meal. Coffee has a heating and stimulating property that allows it to act as a beneficial digesting agent that stimulates the body to effectively break down and assimilate food. The idea of a cup of coffee first thing in the morning on an empty stomach has never been the traditional European way to drink coffee. Coffee (only a small cup, without milk) at the end of a large meal is a functional digestive aid. Europeans feel so strongly about coffee as a digestive aid that they will not drink a latte or cappuccino after a meal because they believe that the milk interferes with coffee's digestive ability. I overheard a waiter in Italy dissuade an American woman from ordering a cappuccino after a large meal. He wouldn't even bring her the cappuccino, only a small shot of espresso.

> **Siesta Time:** In many countries, a small siesta is a traditional opportunity for a walk and a short rest in order to digest the large midday meal. It is not a sleep that lasts the whole afternoon, but a brief respite to focus the body's energy on digestion, instead of mixing up food and work.

The Afternoon Lull

Do you ever notice that in the mid-afternoon you often feel a dip in your energy? This is when many people crave sugar, a cup of coffee, or a jolt of caffeine to boost their energy. In the afternoon, the nervous system cycles in and demands a significant amount of the body's blood sugar. Although we feel the effects of this, the reason behind it is not well known in our culture. Remember that the brain uses up to 80% of the body's blood sugar, and in the afternoon, the brain is demanding its fuel. If you ate only a salad while sitting in front of your computer for lunch, or if your child picked at lunch for 5 to 10 minutes before running to the playground, both of you are left with an empty gas tank. The hungry brain hits the alarm. As far as the body is concerned this is an emergency; the brain requires its fuel in the afternoon just as surely as the sun rises and sets each day. For this reason, Americans find themselves craving chocolate, coffee, candy, soda pop, or a nap in the afternoon.

In Europe it is understood that you don't mess with the midday meal. Many shops still close for an hour or two at midday. It is rare throughout traditional Europe and Asia for the midday meal not to be considered sacred. A satisfying, relaxed lunch helps the body get through the afternoon lull smoothly and efficiently.

Sound the Alarm

When the nervous system is activated in the afternoon and there is no gas in the tank because of an insufficient lunch, a stress-fighting chemistry that has degenerative effects on the body sets in. It begins when the brain sends an emergency message seeking a quick source of energy. A sugar or caffeine craving is a natural physiological response. When kids walk in the front door at three o'clock after having a less than adequate lunch, their brains are in a full-blown emergency response. They will inhale sugar-filled snacks, while their biochemical stress response is moving full steam ahead.

To help the brain get its fuel, the body responds to the stress of low blood sugar and cravings by stimulating the adrenal glands to release stress-fighting hormones, which stimulate the liver to release its stores of glucose into the bloodstream, thereby raising blood sugar. These hormones, though, are degenerative by nature and produce free radicals as waste products. Damaging free radicals are now considered to be the leading cause of aging, disease, cancer, and even death. They oxidize the good cholesterol in the body into bad cholesterol, causing it to adhere to the arterial walls and predisposing people to heart disease. The body is then directed to store all the circulating fat in the bloodstream into fat cells. The same craving that tells the body that it was unable to make it throughout the day on its own without outside support also clearly signals the body not to burn any stored fat for fuel. Until the stressful situation is over, the body continues to send the message: "Store all the available fat under the mattress." Fat is the body's most precious fuel supply.

Fat is burned by the body in a stable, even fashion with no peaks and valleys. A fat-burning system produces stable moods and great endurance. But in times of stress, the body burns the quick and unstable sugar first—and energy and moods destabilize, creating the roller coaster-like effect of blood sugar highs and lows. The fat remains stored by the body until all cravings, stress, and starvation-based diets have been eliminated. Sadly, in our society, because of the pace at which we push ourselves and our children, it is rare that the body ever moves out of the emergency mode of life.

Let's Talk About Obesity

> Obesity is clearly emerging as the leading public health issue of the
> 21st century. —American Obesity Association

The United States of Obesity are on the rise. In the past decade, according to the *Journal of the American Medical Association,* obesity levels have increased in every state—doubling in the past 20 years.

One result these soaring rates is a 30% increase in the reported cases of adult-onset diabetes in the 1990s. This disease, which often develops in overweight adults, is now commonplace in children as young as 10 years old—a sign of the dangerous implications of the rise in nationwide obesity rates.

In France, where there is an obesity rate of only 8%, compared to 33% in America, the diet is one of the richest and highest in fat in the world. French people love butter, but have a surprisingly low level of cardiovascular disease, cholesterol levels, and obesity. How is it that the French can get away with eating such a heavy high-fat diet and not get fat? It may be due to their emphasis on a large midday meal and their lack of snacking.

A study focusing on different eating patterns or habits recorded that the French consumed 60% of their day's calories before two o'clock in the afternoon. The midday meal was followed by a small supper. As a result of eating substantially in the middle of the day, their nervous systems were satisfied throughout the afternoon craving hours. The French follow the Ayurvedic recommendations: breakfast is a piece of baguette or a small croissant, lunch is substantial and satisfying, and the evening meal is small and supplemental. Another study by the Boston University School of Medicine revealed that the French ate less than one snack per day, compared to Americans who snacked at least three times per day. The French are not avoiding snacking as a result of their Herculean willpower; it is simply a result of being satisfied by their large midday meal.

In addition to eating a substantial lunch and light supper, the main meal of the day, as most all the meals in Europe, is enjoyed in a very relaxed, unhurried atmosphere. Offices close down for the lunch hours, people sit and eat leisurely in a park, and a social meal in a restaurant is expected to be eaten at a leisurely pace. Customers are not hurried out the door. It is considered rude in many places to bring the bill before the diners are finished, and people often sit and have a hot drink like an espresso after the meal to aid digestion.

Our typical American hurriedness is a habit that really needs to change. We have to start teaching our children the importance of sitting down together as a family and eating in a relaxed, comfortable environment. Many families sit in front of the TV while they eat their main meal. But it is not only the television; we talk on the phone, drive our car, read our mail, flip through magazines, and work on the computer—all while we are eating. These are bad habits that our children will inherit.

The Healing Power of Slow Food

When I first returned from my postgraduate training in India, I became the co-director of Dr. Deepak Chopra's Health Center in Boston, where I stayed for eight years and treated a range of people for many health problems, including cancer and other terminal illnesses. I designed treatment programs, diets, and exercise routines. People would typically come and spend a week at the center to get their life back on track. During a given week, people were bombarded with information and knowledge to help empower them mentally and emotionally to get well.

At the end of their week, they were asked: "What was the most important thing you learned during your week at the Health Center?"

I was completely surprised to hear the same answer over and over again. The most common response people gave was that they realized for the first time that eating was not a filling station, where you drive up, inhale the fuel, and speed off.

These people were starting to recognize the importance of sitting down in a relaxed fashion and digesting a well-cooked meal. They never realized that eating could be such a pleasurable experience. Because there were so many powerful treatments and educational programs they were exposed to at the Center, hearing person after person say that sitting down and eating a relaxed meal was the most most important thing they learned was a profound eye-opener.

With that in mind, parents have to make that special effort to bring the family together, sit down, and have a relaxed meal. Yes, I am asking parents to consider eating a larger midday meal and a smaller sit-down family soup-like supper early in the evening if possible. I'll share how we do it in our home.

Our Daily Routine

Breakfast

We usually start the day sitting down at the breakfast table with hot cereal, fruits or eggs, and toast. The goal of this meal is for it to be large enough for the children and ourselves to be able to make it to lunchtime without cravings. At this meal we serve our children each an 8-ounce glass of water that they are required to drink. (If we don't put mandatory water into their routine, they may rarely drink it.)

Lunch

The lunchtime meal at school for the children comes with the instruction, "do the best you can," with all the encouragement and convincing to finish their lunch that we can possibly muster. We take the time to make their lunch, so we are slightly attached to them eating it, even though that may be about 50% of the time.

My wife and I have a substantial meal together at around one o'clock, either meeting at a restaurant for lunch or eating a meal she has prepared at home. This is our most important meal of the day.

After School

The food from lunch sits on the stove till around three o'clock, slightly warm, until the kids walk in the door—starving!!! Fortunately, there is some warm, healthful food with vegetables waiting. We simply put it in front of them and watch it disappear. This is like magic compared to trying to force-feed them at dinner. Often, if my wife and I have eaten lunch at a restaurant, we will order some take-out to bring home so the kids will have some cooked, wholesome food waiting for them when they get home from school.

Homework or Playtime

Now the kids' nervous systems have a full tank of gas—the brain is not craving sugar or producing a degenerative chemistry, and the body is not storing fat. The brain is stable, moods are stable, and the chaos and pandemonium that we otherwise experience are gone. The kids get along, they don't complain about doing their homework, and most importantly, they're not bouncing off the walls!

Supper

At around six or seven in the evening we sit down all together and share a small family supper. My wife and I are still quite content from our midday meal. This is primarily a social gathering to connect with the children, rather than a feeding time for Mom and Dad. We may have a bowl of soup and a piece of toast for supper, while the kids have something more substantial (children often require three square meals a day). At this time the children are not in a major blood sugar low nor have they declared war on their vegetables. They are stable, and eating seems to be an acceptable behavior.

I wish I could say our family runs this smoothly every single day, but it is the general theme of what happens in our home. When we tried eating they way most Americans do, we found life became exhaustingly chaotic and stressful.

Remember the 51% Rule

When I make recommendations to encourage a family to alter their lifestyle, I realize that these changes are difficult to make. I don't expect parents to turn their entire family routine upside down because they read a chapter in this book. When I first started using these principles, I used the 51% rule. I strove to follow this lifestyle 51% of the time, so that I lived the majority of my life by going with the flow and moving with the cycles of nature.

The impact of a weekly routine that involves five days of getting up early and two of sleeping in will provide the benefit of getting up early the majority of the time. Drinking coffee occasionally has a significantly milder impact on the body than consuming a whole pot each day. It's easy to see that the habits we follow the majority of the time are the ones which set the tone for our lives.

Commit to a trial period of change and give it three or four days a week. You'll quickly notice the difference and experience the benefits of this change. You may adjust the other days to fit into this more natural lifestyle. When you do something that makes you feel good, it's usually a just matter of time before it becomes a way of life.

The Blood Sugar Roller Coaster

Every parent has witnessed a child experiencing low blood sugar. When the blood sugar roller coaster takes a plunge, the child's moods and energy often go with it. A hungry, cranky baby is just trying to communicate that blood sugar is low. If your child seems moody or depressed, has attention deficit concerns, and he or she is constantly craving sugar or caffeine, then your child is glued to the out-of-control roller coaster seat. When the roller coaster is up and the blood sugar is high, the mood is great. When the roller coaster dips down and the blood sugar is low, the mood and energy are low. This child has lost control of his or her mood.

Remember, the roller coaster stimulates the production and release of degenerative stress-fighting hormones, discharging disease-producing free radicals, causing fat storage, continual sweet cravings, and anxiety, fatigue, exhaustion, and depression. The longer this continues, the more all of these effects will continue to spiral out of control. This is a powerful set-up for teenagers, who, in reaction to this stress, often reach out to the wrong crowd to self-medicate problems away. Cigarettes, drugs, and alcohol are common coping mechanisms for an uncontrolled blood sugar roller coaster.

Lifestyle Study

As I have emphasized, it is your consistent choice—what you do

51% of the time, or in the majority of your life—that can have either the most rejuvenating or the most degenerative effects on your body. If you are doing good things for yourself regularly, the results will be very favorable. But an unbalanced lifestyle followed consistently will be severely degenerative.

The lifestyle I am recommending is not something radical; it was the original American way of life. To illustrate to others the power of this lifestyle, I conducted a preliminary study based on the concepts of my book, *The 3-Season Diet.* The basic premise of the study was to measure the effect of eating a large lunch and a light dinner on weight loss. I also measured the effect of this lifestyle change on other maladies including: levels of anxiety, depression, cravings, insomnia, fatigue, after-work exhaustion, and people's general sense of well-being. All of these conditions improved significantly in only two weeks without the use of any additional drugs or herbal medicines. Even though I measured an adult population, the results were powerful and lend credibility to the lifestyle routine I'm recommending you embrace for your whole family's optimal health.

Weight Loss and Lifestyle Study Summary

My study measured the effects of specific lifestyle changes on the following common complaints that plague average Americans. Twenty subjects were recruited for the two-month study, which was advertised as a weight-loss lifestyle study.

My colleagues and I did not eliminate interested participants from the study for any reason, so we had many individuals in the group who were taking medications for serious conditions including: diabetes, depression, high blood pressure, and asthma, as well as hormone replacement therapy. Considering that many of our participants were generally unhealthy and taking pharmaceutical medications, many of which had side effects including weight gain, only lends higher credibility to the results we would have seen in a healthy population. This study, however, does reflect accurate and predictable results for the average overweight American.

The participants were asked to eat a moderate breakfast, a

large, healthful, and satisfying lunch at midday, and then to attempt to have only water in the evening. If they were uncomfortable or developed food cravings, they were told to eat a light supper, like a soup or salad. Exercise with nasal breathing and seasonal eating were suggested but not emphasized in the study.

Maximum levels of weight loss and increase in the sense of well-being in all subjective measures were expected to occur when only two meals a day—breakfast and lunch—were eaten with copious amounts of water and herb tea for dinner for the full seven days per week. The participants were able to consume only water for dinner an average of three and a half days out of seven.

There were some members in the group who complained of severe blood sugar disorders, who before participating in the study had a hard time limiting themselves to three meals a day without suffering severe cravings or side effects. The fact that they were conditioned to eat every two hours meant that participating in this study was a dramatic shift in their behavior. As the weeks went by, all the study participants noticed that they were able to eat less for dinner; almost all of them reached the point of being able to consume only water for dinner two to three times a week. This is a powerful testimonial for the effect that living life with nature's rhythms has on physiological processes like the stabilization of the blood sugar roller coaster. As the participants' energy and blood sugar levels became more stable, they reported dramatic improvements in levels of anxiety, depression, fatigue, cravings, and in the quality of their sleep.

During the 8-week study, the participants were able to lose a healthy average of 1.2 pounds per week. If they were to follow this program for one year at that level of weight loss, it would represent a significant weight loss of 62.4 pounds per year. To measure their levels of improvement in their other health concerns, they self-reported changes based on a subjective questionnaire. The changes that they reported were significant.

For more precise details about the results of this study, feel free to contact me via the Internet at: info@lifespa.com.

The advantage of introducing these lifestyle recommendations when your children are young is that it will be easier for them to incorporate this supportive schedule into their lifestyle while they are still developing their habits and patterns. If you can teach them to flow downstream with the current when they are young, they can avoid the toll that decades of rowing upstream can take on their health.

The Current American Schedule of Eating Is Not Working

The average American is overweight, and a significant proportion of the population complains of fatigue, cravings, anxiety, and depression. America is the fattest country in the world, with the highest levels of chronic disease. In this study, we strove to show that a simple and sustainable change in lifestyle could change the causative factors of many of the chronic conditions plaguing Americans without the use of drugs, medicine, surgery, or a rigid starvation diet. Our discoveries support the idea that just by changing our schedules to flow with the current, we can noticeably improve our health and well-being. Adults and children can follow these lifestyle suggestions with important benefits for their health.

Natural Weight Balancing

When I was a kid, we ate supper at around 5:30 every night. This was very common; in fact many other kids ate even earlier than five o'clock. By six o'clock, we were all back out on the streets playing kick-the-can, basketball, or the game of the night. By nine o'clock we were back inside, in the shower, and off to bed. We woke up around 6:30 the next morning and were eating breakfast by seven. We didn't think about the fact that we were fasting from six o'clock in the evening until seven o'clock the following morning. That's 13 hours! During this natural fasting experience the body is forced to burn fat as fuel, so by morning it was time to break the fast with a delicious, light, and aptly named "break-fast" meal.

Fasting each night resets the body's ability to burn fat as a stable fuel source. By doing this for a significant period of each day (13 hours), we had the freedom to eat as much sugar as we wanted during the day. Not that sugar is good in any way, but our sugar intake was unrestricted and we used it on just about everything. In spite of that, it was rare to hear of anyone complaining about blood sugar issues, mood problems, energy fluctuations, weight gain, or difficulty with attention.

American culture advocates eating meals every two to three hours to help stabilize blood sugar levels. This will certainly keep the highs and lows of the roller coaster from becoming too intense and will temporarily prop up the blood sugar level. With this style of eating, the body becomes accustomed to going from one carbohydrate meal to another and learns how to survive from sugar meal to sugar meal. This results in the need to de-condition the body from its inability to make energy last for more than a few hours. When I was a kid, our natural nighttime fast reset fat metabolism, a stable source of fuel that provided a baseline of constant energy throughout the day. Although the sugar we ate was surely not good for us, it didn't create the roller coaster ride we see today due to the baseline of stable fat-burning metabolism that would not let our blood sugar dip dangerously low. This seems like a simple concept, and it is unfortunate that it has been largely forgotten.

Eating really should be so simple. The basic rules for eating to maintain good health and proper weight are:

Breakfast is a large enough meal to last you until lunchtime without cravings.

Lunch is a large enough meal to last you until suppertime without cravings.

Supper is a large enough meal, preferably taken as early as possible, to last you until bedtime without cravings.

All meals are relaxed and unhurried.
If possible, do not snack.

Could that be simpler?

Treating Childhood Obesity

The following is a method for treating childhood obesity by encouraging the body to sustain a fat-burning metabolism. These rules, modified for children, are step-by-step instructions that have proven to stabilize moods and energy and to reduce weight in children.

Instructions

Before Breakfast: Morning exercise before breakfast sustains energy throughout the day.

Breakfast: Eat fruit. (If unable to sustain energy on just fruit, add small portions of toast, cereal, or eggs.) Breakfast needs to be large enough to last until lunch without hunger pangs.

Lunch: The largest meal of the day. This can be right after school. For the school lunch meal, eat enough to comfortably last until the after-school lunch meal. The large meal could be something like rice, chicken, vegetables, salad, soup, dessert, and water. It should be large, complete, and satisfying. For the body to digest this substantial meal it is necessary to relax while eating and rest for 5 to 10 minutes after eating before going back to your day. Relax. Don't watch TV, open mail, drive, ride in the car, or talk on the phone.

Supper (Supplemental—before six o'clock is ideal): This is the most important time of the day to re-educate the body to burn fat for energy rather than relying on and craving sugars, breads, and carbohydrates. Remember, this meal needs to be large enough to last until bedtime without hunger. But this process should be effortless. If you find yourself straining in order not to eat, then the body's emergency response will kick in and trigger cravings for more sugar (emergency fuel) and store the very fat you are trying to burn.

Implementation of the program is by phases. Move from the first phase to the second or third only if it feels effortless to do so and there are no cravings. Otherwise, revert back to a previous phase.

Phase 1: Eat soup, salad, or fruit for supper. This will be easy if the lunch meal is large, relaxed, and satisfying. Start out with a

> **Make sure to drink enough water to stay fully hydrated!**

more substantial supper if you aren't going to bed comfortable. As the blood sugar stabilizes over the first couple of weeks, the ability to reduce the size of supper will naturally improve.

For more significant weight loss, it is possible to progress directly from Phase 1 to Phase 3. Certain kid-types will not be able to progress beyond Phase 1 or 2. Encourage your child to listen to their bodies carefully. The ability to progress is determined by the ease with which the child can sustain his or her energy.

Water Break: If meals are eaten as recommended, hunger pangs may be thirst. Drink 8 to 10 ounces of water when a hunger pang hits and wait 10 minutes. If hunger persists, have a small snack.

Phase 2: If Phase 1 feels easy and comfortable, then after five o'clock take in only liquids (fruit or vegetable juice, broth, herb tea with honey).If cravings persist, drink more water and have a larger and more relaxed lunch. If this isn't working, go back to Phase 1.

Phase 3: Once Phases 1 and 2 are established effortlessly, drink 3 to 6 liters of water from lunch to breakfast the following morning. Drinking herb tea with honey in the evening is okay. To offset hunger pangs, drink 8 ounces of water every hour or two from lunch until bedtime. Phase 3 allows the body to fast from lunch to "breakfast" the next morning, forcing the body to burn fat for energy.

> Try to stay on Phase 2 or 3 for at least four weeks for optimal results. Remember: if your child cannot easily perform any of these phases, then follow a regime of three square meals a day. Slowly and gracefully, your child's blood sugar will start to stabilize, and he or she will be able to make longer trips between meals without cravings. In the beginning, use Phases 1, 2, and 3 interchangeably as needed to keep the blood sugar stable.

Eating Seasonally

On the 3-Season Diet Grocery List in Chapter 7, circle the foods you like for each season and then, during that season, eat as much as you like of those foods. Think in terms of what foods you can eat a lot of and don't think of any food as a bad food. There is not a "do not eat" list, just a list of foods that are better to eat when in season. (In nature, when cherries are in season, the birds eat nothing but cherries for three to four weeks.) If it is in season and you like it, give yourself permission to eat as much of it as you like. Just stop for the day by six o'clock in the evening.

Remember

This program is designed to allow the body to utilize fat as an energy source and reduce unnatural cravings for sugar. In the beginning it may be difficult for your child to make this transition from a dependency on sugar to a stable fat-burning metabolism, so use Phases 1, 2, and 3 interchangeably until it becomes effortless. If you feed your child a large lunch and he or she doesn't feel hungry in the evening, then try Phase 3 the following day. But if their evening hunger persists, follow Phase 1 or 2. By working with the body it soon will become easy to follow Phase 2 or 3 for weeks at a time and metabolize stored fat. Once your child is able to establish a desired weight, then that weight can be effortlessly maintained by following a Phase 1 approach or by enjoying a light evening meal. Once in a while, your child can enjoy a big dinner because he or she will be learn to balance a larger dinner with a light lunch.

 Remember, it is what you do every day that will make a difference. For further details see *The 3-Season Diet.*

Botanical Support

In some cases a child or adult will simply not be able to make it from a Phase 1 to a Phase 2 regimen even after following the program for a couple of weeks. In the lifestyle study, the participants noticed that the longer they were on the program, the easier it was make their energy last into the evening. Slowly, by working with their body and not forcing themselves to do anything they felt uncomfortable with, the group was able to progress naturally from Phase 1 to Phase 3.

In certain cases, when the blood sugar has been strained for an extended period of time there can be a need for botanical support to help strengthen the pancreas.

Gurmar

The most effective herb for strengthening pancreatic functions is called *gurmar* (Sugar Destroyer) or *shardunika*.

- Botanical Name: *Gymnema sylvestre*
- Botany: A climbing plant found in central and southern India
- Parts Used: Root and leaves
- Chemistry: The leaves and roots are rich in gymnemic acids or triterpine saponins. These are acids that contain a complex mixture of at least 9 glycosides, which are acidic plant sugars.
- Action: diuretic, astringent, stomachic, and tonic. Lowers blood sugar levels in hyperglycemic individuals but, amazingly, has no effect on people with normal blood sugar. Decreases sugar cravings.
- Indications: Glycosuria (sugar in the urine), urinary disorders, sugar sensitivities, and diabetes. Studies have shown that gurmar increases the ability of Islet of Langerhans cells in the pancreas to secrete insulin in people who have either type I or type II diabetes.

How To Take Gurmar:
This herb is best taken in 500 milligram doses, in capsules, one half hour before meals. It is still effective if taken right before meals or even after meals.

Gymnema will help stop sugar cravings throughout the day, and most importantly it will stabilize both high and low blood sugar levels. People who have become severely sugar-intolerant can reintroduce moderate doses of sugar back into their diet after taking this herb for two to six months. For children who have overdone their sugar consumption and are unable to move from Phase 1 to Phase 2, or simply cannot follow Phase 1 without severe cravings, gymnema is an extremely important herb to resolve their blood sugar instability.

The River of Life

When your boat is pointed downstream with the current, life seems to be going your way, but most of us live life paddling upstream and find ourselves and our family exhausted at the end of each day. The flow of this current is reflected in our bodies through our natural inclination to eat, sleep, exercise, and even think at different and unique times of day. Some of these suggestions may be impossible for your family. That's fine. Just take the ones that work for you and implement them using the 51% rule. When you have just a taste of the results of a living a life that flows downstream, paddling upstream again becomes unthinkable. I remember one patient who put it so perfectly:

> *Once you start this program it is very difficult to go back to the old ways—because you felt so lousy. So I guess I'm stuck feeling good.*
> —L. Martin

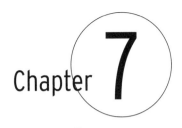

Chapter 7

Secret 6—For Each Season There Is a Reason

H ave you ever wondered why squirrels eat nuts in the winter? Why birds can't get enough of those delicious cherries in the spring? Or why nature makes such an abundance of apples in the fall? Maybe there is some truth to the old saying, "An apple a day keeps the doctor away," or maybe the birds and squirrels know something we don't.

For the past 50 years the debate over high-protein, low-fat, and high-carbohydrate diets has been confusing and contradictory. Each diet is backed by convincing scientific research arguing that it is the best and only way to eat properly and lose weight. Each diet promises the same benefits: more energy, better stamina, weight loss, and an improved sense of well-being. But how can they all be right?

The answer is astonishingly simple. Each one *is* right, but for only four months of the year! The secret to making these different diets work together over a lifetime is to use each one in the appropriate season: low-fat in the spring, high-carbohydrate in the summer, and high-fat and protein-rich in the winter. The three-season approach aligns our desires with the seasonal foods that have been provided by nature for thousands of years.

If we pay attention to our cravings as they change throughout the year, we will notice that in the winter we naturally crave soups, nuts, warm grains, meat, and fish. These high-fat and protein-rich foods help warm the body and insulate it from cold. In the spring, we feel drawn to salads, berries, and leafy greens—a low-fat diet to help burn off the weight stored to keep us warm during the cold winter months. And in the summer, when the days are long and hot, we most enjoy high-energy foods that have a cooling action—the in-season high-carbohydrate fruits and vegetables.

Even though we generally talk about the four seasons of the year—winter, spring, summer, and fall—three of these are primary growing and harvesting seasons, and one is a season of rest. The harvests are in the spring, summer, and fall; the season of rest is the dormant winter. We eat spring and summer harvests in the season they are harvested, while the fall harvest stretches through both the fall and winter, giving us a three-season approach to eating.

What Should Kids Eat?

The debate about the best foods for an adult to eat is confusing enough, let alone what to feed children. The barrage of information and all the media coverage of different diets have not helped Americans lose weight. Even with our emphasis on restrictive diets, 65% of Americans are overweight. Inevitably, some of the extreme and restrictive weight-loss eating styles have overflowed onto our children's plates. In this chapter, I will describe a simple and logical approach to eating for both children and adults that gracefully restores the balance that once existed in the American diet.

I want to be clear that in no way am I suggesting that children, or adults for that matter, go on a diet. Diets don't work; they never have and never will. The three-season approach to eating outlined in this chapter is not a weight-loss diet involving good and bad foods, calorie counting, tasteless meals, low-fat substitutes, willpower, and restrictions. I am not suggesting you only eat foods that are in season, but to eat more of those seasonal foods. By eating increased amounts of foods that are in season, the medicinal benefits of seasonal foods are enjoyed, cravings are reduced, and the lost connection to the local farmer is gracefully restored. For most people this becomes a preferred way of life rather than a diet.

At the end of this chapter there is a kid-friendly grocery list for each season: fall/winter, summer, and spring. This shopping list is a grocery store decoder. At a glance, parents can choose the foods that are in season in order to glean the benefits of eating with nature's cycles. Remember, the goal is not to adhere rigidly to a seasonal grocery list. It is to enjoy more seasonal foods by shifting the emphasis of in-season foods throughout the year. Of course, you can eat out-of-season foods as long as you are eating an abundance of the food nature is intending during that season. Parents will realize that seasonal foods are the ones that they naturally crave and prefer.

> **No bad foods:** There are no completely bad foods; there are only foods that are better for you when they are in season.

There Is More to Food Than Calories

In Europe, where cardiovascular disease and obesity levels are extremely low, the cuisine is regarded by many to be the world's best. The Mediterranean diet, touted for its great-tasting food, gained notoriety in the early 1990s when Dr. Ancel Keys at the University of Minnesota measured the diet's ability to reduce the risk of heart disease and prevent many common cancers.

Mediterranean countries value eating and coming together for a meal as important parts of the social culture. Fresh and seasonal foods are purchased daily from local markets. There are different shops for vegetables, breads, meats, fish, cheese, and wine. People stay connected to their local farmers naturally and effortlessly.

> We tend of think of diet only in terms of how many proteins, fats, and carbohydrates we ingest. But there is much more to our food than numbers. Enjoying our food and eating seasonally provide benefits that go beyond the paint-by-numbers approach of calorie counting.

Diets: A No No

If you come across a diet plan that includes a group of forbidden foods, I suggest that you run the other way as fast as you can. These diets are bound to fail because human nature makes us want what we cannot have. If you tell your children that they cannot eat candy or watch TV, they may follow that rule for a while, but soon the cravings for candy and TV will become so strong that they will, by hook or by crook, find a way to obtain what was taken away.

Researchers found that mice put on diets also binge on forbidden foods when given the chance. Studies done with mice at the Massachusetts Institute of Technology showed that restrictive diets don't work for this reason. Researchers fed mice a high-protein and high-fat diet for an extended period of time and then measured weight loss. Without adequate carbohydrates, the mice were forced to obtain their energy from fat cells—and lost weight as a result. When the mice were put back on an unrestricted diet and carbohydrates were available, they binged, gaining all the lost weight back and then some. Low-carbohydrate diets are a brilliant technique to force the body into fat metabolism. The only problem is that the body is under such duress in the process that it needs to recover, so it rebounds—with a few extra pounds of insurance.

Remember in the last chapter I talked about the body's response to stress? The first response is to put the fat under the body's mattress (the fat cells) and store it until the body is convinced that the emergency or siege is over. When you force the body to burn fat by removing energy-rich carbohydrates or fats from the diet, it is only a matter of time before uncontrollable cravings and binging set in.

> The problem with restricting foods as a technique for balancing energy and moods and losing weight is that our predicted physiological response to deprivation is to crave what is missing and then binge on those restricted foods.

According to research done by the National Institutes of Health, 99% of people who go on diets regain every pound they lose within three to five years.

Winter Wisdom

In the dry and cold winter season, there is a tendency for the body to also become dry and cold. Of course, this can vary depending on an individual's body type. For example, Sarah, a winter—or Vata—kid-type, lives in Montana and in January she is a cold kid in a cold climate. If she eats a lot of cold foods such as salad and dry rice cakes or crackers, and drinks milkshakes, ice tea, and cold soda pop, she will begin to develop problems related to excessive cold. Sarah's blood vessels will be constricted, causing dry tissues, constipation, dry skin, poor circulation (making Sarah feel even colder), and dehydration. By now you know that children are in the spring lifecycle and that they react to dryness by making excessive mucus. This mucus is a perfect breeding ground for opportunistic bacterial and viral infections. By becoming excessively dry and chronically dehydrated, Sarah is setting herself up for winter colds and flus, spring allergies, and battles with a runny nose.

> Diets may work at first but they will later fail. Eating seasonally is our best diet. There are no absolute restrictions because there are no bad foods; there are just foods which are better for you when they are in season.

Squirrels know better than to try to subsist on salads in the winter the way Sarah does. They eat a diet favoring high-protein and fat-packed nuts, which are part of nature's fall harvest. Other foods in this natural fall harvest are whole grains. These are generally thought of as a high-carbohydrate food, but they are filled with healthy oils and proteins. These warm, insulating foods of the fall harvest are nature's attempts to remedy the drying action of this season on the skin and sinuses. One of the hallmarks of the Mediterranean diet is the high-quality fat content in their low-meat, high-nut, grain, and seed, and vegetable-based diet. These high-fat, high-protein foods are the perfect antidote to the cold-aggravating properties of the winter season.

Even in Hawaii or other tropical climates, foods with a higher fat and protein content are naturally more abundant in the winter.

Some of these abundant foods are the cold-water fish that migrate to tropical waters in the winter. These fish provide the local people with a source of warm and insulating marine oils high in essential fatty acids (EFAs): the omega-3 and omega-6 fatty acids. Far from causing obesity, these good winter fats provide a sense of satiety in the diet, helping to prevent the overeating that can lead to weight gain, and lowering the circulating cholesterol that will compromise even a child's cardiovascular system. (I will discuss EFAs in more detail in Chapter 10.)

According to Ayurveda, winter is the season in which the body most effectively stores proteins, fats, minerals, and vitamins. A nutrient-rich winter diet builds the body's reserves for the remainder of the year. If a diet rich in these nutrients is not eaten in the winter, then the reserves that give the body energy and stamina throughout the spring and summer will be depleted. As winter moves into spring, throughout March and April, an unsatisfied body is set up for cravings, blood sugar highs and lows, weight gain, and mood instability.

Parental Tip: If the body does not capitalize on winter's ability to store proteins and fats, these deficiencies will sow the seeds of imbalance in the months and years to come. Make sure your child is eating more nuts, seeds, grains, and meats in the winter months.

The Skinny on Fat

Americans must forget the idea that fats are bad. Fats are a compact, high-energy source of food. Gram for gram, fats provide twice the energy of carbohydrates. Up to two-thirds of the total energy for the cells may be supplied by fats. If fats are eaten excessively or if the body is under a lot of stress, the body will store energy in fat cells along with unused carbohydrates and proteins. But fats essential functions in the body, making them an integral component of a healthy diet.

Low-Fat Doesn't Mean Low-Calorie!

It is a good idea to avoid feeding children processed low-fat foods. Many of these low-fat foods actually pack more calories then their full-fat or natural counterparts. The National Heart, Lung, and Blood Institute Obesity Guidelines urge you to read labels and compare calories. Here are some surprising examples: a fat-free fig cookie has 70 calories, while a regular one has only 50. A 1/2 cup serving of nonfat ice cream or frozen yogurt yields 10 calories more than the regular version. Experts agree that the practice of reducing all fats in the name of good health can easily backfire. It can result in an increased caloric intake resulting in more obese children and a population-wide deficiency in the beneficial and essential fats that offer a baseline of stable energy for the body.

Winter Rest

The long nights and short days of winter are nature's way of insisting we take more rest. During these months, the body's metabolic rate naturally slows down, encouraging rest even for those animals, like ourselves, who do not hibernate. This rest allows the body to store the energy and high-quality nutrients that will be drawn on in the spring and summer. In order to allow children to build up their reserves, it is important to get them to bed early in the winter. Most of the time a child's illnesses during cold and flu season can be traced to being run down. A combination of after-school activities, increased academic responsibilities, and social pressures can be more than enough to deplete children's reserves and make them susceptible to a cold or flu. I think that most parents would agree that when their child gets sick, they can often trace the cause to exhaustion, fatigue, and over-scheduling in their child's life.

Although adults may be able to push their limits, children have much less resiliency. In our home, we do our best to get the children, particularly the younger ones, to bed by eight o'clock. I cannot over-emphasize the importance of keeping your child properly rested. In the summertime, when there is no school and the days are longer, the sleep schedule does not have to be as strict.

But during cold and flu season, the best method of protecting a child against a cold or flu just might be the right amount of rest. I should mention that going to bed late and sleeping in late into the morning does not provide the same benefits as going to bed early. The longer a person lies in bed in the morning, as I mentioned in Chapter 6, the sleepier, duller, and more lethargic they will become.

Imagine going to bed at midnight and getting up at ten o'clock in the morning? How would you feel compared to going to bed at eight o'clock and getting up at six in the morning? Most people feel that if they did the latter, they would feel more rejuvenated, whereas they'd feel tired and dull if they got up at ten. The difference is when the sleep occurred. Although both nights' sleep lasted exactly ten hours, there is a dramatic difference in the quality of rest and energy in the morning. The hours from ten at night until two in the morning are the hours of metabolic cleansing and renewal in the body, and sleeping at this time brings the most rest to the entire body.

Are You Ready for Spring?

Winter dryness leads to spring mucus. The steps you take in the winter to reduce dryness will pay dividends in the spring. As parents, you will soon begin to see how your child's health, or lack thereof, can be traced to the imbalances created a season or two prior. Letting the body dry out in the winter will only increase the risk of developing allergies and other mucus-related conditions in the spring.

Spring is characterized by high humidity, frequent rain, wet and congested earth, temperatures transitioning from cold to warm, germinating seeds, and growing plants. This is the time of the most austere harvest of the year, rich only in sprouts, leafy greens, mushrooms, grapefruits and other citrus fruits, and some roots and berries. All of these foods are naturally low in fat, and in many cases they have natural fat-burning properties. Remember the grapefruit diets? They were heralded as miracle diets due to the fat-emulsifying properties of grapefruit. It is not a coincidence that grapefruit is harvested in the spring when these properties are needed.

Most of all, foods harvested in the spring are dry and serve as an antidote to the season's mucus-producing rains and humidity. Not following a spring diet can have significant consequences for a child. If a spring kid-type in the spring lifecycle, like 9-year-old James, who is prone to colds and frequent sinus congestion and earaches, eats a diet full of pizza, cold soda pop, and ice cream in late March, he will produce excess mucus. A scenario like this sets up that all-too-familiar situation of compromised lymphatic circulation and drainage, which inhibits an appropriate immune response combined with a rich, stagnant breeding ground for bacterial and viral infections. Nature's antidote to this dilemma is simply the harvest at hand.

Secret 6: No More Diets: The sixth secret is to eat the foods provided by the harvest of the season. There is a relationship between foods and the time of year they ripen naturally. Each harvest offers medicinal benefits to protect us from that season's maladies. Eating seasonally provides us with the changing nutritional requirements we need for the vastly different times of the year.

Backyard Medicines

Not even a hundred years ago, leafy greens and root vegetables were a mainstay of the American diet. Dandelions, for example, were not Backyard Enemy Number One, but a dependable food source that offered important health benefits. Dandelion tea was a common drink in every household. It provided a natural diuretic to enhance circulation and remove stagnation and impurities from the blood and lymph. Its tender greens pop up in the humid spring season when they are needed to remove the excess water from the body.

Other backyard medicines are the rhizomes or surface roots of plants, which deer and other animals uncover when the snows begin to melt and the ground softens. The animals chew these bitter and astringent roots throughout the spring to remove excess mucus from the intestinal tract. These rhizomes are rich in bitter chemicals that are known to cleanse the blood and detoxify the deep tissues of

> It is amazing to realize how nature has provided protection for our health through its seasonal harvests. The roots and rhizomes eaten in early spring remove the excess mucus that could act as a breeding ground for bad bacteria. Once the excess mucus is removed, right on cue, nature provides the perfect fertilizer for good bacteria in the form of chlorophyll-rich greens and sprouts.

the body. The rhizomes that were once part of the American diet are still a mainstay in the natural world. Sadly, we have lost the tradition of using these rhizomes, roots, and leafy greens in our diet.

If we continue to watch what deer or other animals eat, we see that once the excess mucus of spring is properly balanced by seasonally harvested rhizomes, they begin to feed on the sprouts that are just beginning to emerge from the ground. These sprouts are rich in easily absorbed chlorophyll, minerals, and trace elements. Chlorophyll is used in the body as a fertilizer to grow beneficial bacteria in the intestinal tract. If we do not eat adequate amounts of sprouts or leafy greens in the spring we run the risk of not properly fertilizing the intestines. As a result, intestinal flora will be disturbed, parasites and pathogenic or bad bacteria can flourish, and out-of-balance yeast overgrowth can thrive. The assimilation of food and nutrients will be compromised, and the health of the child will soon be affected. To prevent or remedy this situation, look at the spring diet at the end of this chapter and eat as many of the greens on the list as possible. Buy or grow lots of sprouts from alfalfa, beans, and almost any nut or seed. If you put them on salads and sandwiches, kids will usually eat them without fuss.

The "Fast" Track

Spring was historically a time for fasting. Jesus fasted in the spring. This is when Native Americans went on (and still go on) vision quests requiring many days of fasting. Other traditional cultures also observe a variety of spring fasting practices. It is natural to fast in the spring when food is scarce, before the spring greens have sprouted. For traditional people fasting was the perfect solution to stretch out a food supply that was running low.

Fasting forces the body into a fat-burning metabolism. This allows the body to burn off some of the excess stored fat from the winter months. It is an even more important opportunity to reset the body's baseline ability to burn its own fat as a primary fuel supply. In the spring, when the body is forced to burn its fat stores, a natural detoxification occurs. The spring-harvested foods provide a diet that is austere and low-fat by nature, including cleansing rhizomes and green vegetables to support detoxification.

In the winter, if adequate amounts of proteins and fats have not been stored, or the body has been chronically dehydrated, the naturally occurring, fat-burning detoxification of the spring will be derailed. Remember the rule: if the body is under stress it will do everything it can to store fat. We are familiar with the results of this chronic stress and lack of seasonal detoxification in America: children are overweight, they do not have a stable fat-burning baseline metabolism, and they live on a diet filled with sugar that yields short-term energy.

When the body is primarily burning fat while fasting, hunger pangs generally disappear. Energy becomes stable and thoughts of food can often be dismissed for days as long as the body stays adequately hydrated. The ability to burn fat as a stable source of fuel is the key to mood stability and a sustainable level of high energy. There are many opportunities throughout the course of the day and during the year to reset your children's fat burning metabolism.

It is not necessary to follow every one of these fat-burning techniques—but it is important to know about them and to use them whenever possible.

Let's review some of the fat-burning opportunities we have discussed so far:

- Exercise first thing in the morning.
- Drink one-half your body weight in ounces of water each day.
- Break the nighttime fast with breakfast.

- Eat a big lunch, or a substantial after-school meal.
- Eat a breakfast large enough to get to lunch without cravings.
- Eat a lunch large enough to get to supper without cravings.
- Eat a supper large enough to get to bedtime without cravings.
- Close the kitchen as early as possible, preferably finishing supper by six o'clock.
- Select the majority of your foods from the spring grocery lists during spring.
- Choose a diet rich in fats and proteins to store adequate amounts of these nutrients during the winter months.
- Increase the amount of exercise or activity in the spring as compared to the winter.

Nature's pH Balance

When you look at a valley of new growth in the spring, the foliage is a bright and vibrant green not seen in any other season. This intense color comes from the leaves of green plants—especially rich in chlorophyll during the spring. Chlorophyll is beneficial to the body because it helps to balance the intestinal flora and provides a cleansing alkaline chemical in the diet.

Beans are some of the seeds that begin to sprout in the warmth and moisture of April and May after lying dormant all winter. As seeds, the beans lie on the ground in the winter, and animals rarely feed on them. Beans are hard to digest because they have hard shells and are very acidic in nature. (Unless they are boiled for several hours, they can be extremely difficult for a child to digest.) In nature, animals eat beans after they begin to sprout in the spring. As a sprout, their nutritional content is up to 400 times more potent than it is as a full-grown plant or as the bean itself. As a sprout, the bean is also transformed, as if by magic, from an acidic to an alkaline food.

All foods are either predominantly acidic or alkaline. Generally, alkaline foods are cleansing, detoxifying, and better for one's health, while acid foods tend to taste better and have a building effect on the body (as long as they are not eaten to excess). The acid-alkaline recommendations suggest that one-third of our diet should be acid-based and two-thirds of the diet alkaline-based. Some common alkaline foods are fruits and vegetables. Common acidic foods are meats, dairy, grains, and sugar (all our comfort foods).

Interestingly, if we look at nature's harvest, we will see that the majority of the acidic foods we eat are part of the fall harvest to be eaten in the cold fall and winter months. These comfort foods are rich in protein and fat, and are extremely important building and insulating foods for optimal health and growth of your child. Come spring and summer, the harvest changes to predominantly alkaline fruits and vegetables.If you simply follow the recommendations of this chapter and eat more of the foods that are in season, you will naturally have a diet that is one-third acid and two-thirds alkaline.

> In nature, the nutritional cycle is an annual cycle. From nature's point of view, it is impossible to take in all the required proteins, fats, and carbohydrates every day of the year as the RDA suggests. Animals gracefully shift their diet from a higher intake of protein and fat in the winter to a lower-fat cleansing diet in the spring and then to a very high fruit and vegetable, carbohydrate-based, energy-rich diet in the summer.

The Green Machine

Colonies of beneficial bacteria live in our intestinal tract. These symbiotic bacteria provide an environment that allows for the proper absorption and breakdown of our food, and they also manufacture necessary nutrients like Vitamin K. If the environment in the intestinal tract becomes too acidic, these bacteria will die off, providing space for bacteria, yeast, or parasites to flourish. An imbalance of intestinal flora, particularly in children, can easily go unnoticed. Frequent use of antibiotics can also lead to death of beneficial bacteria and disruption of natural flora, making room for growth of the undesirables. Excessive yeast, bad bacteria, and parasites can compromise assimilation of food and create bloating, gas, and abdominal pain.

Nature, as I am sure you will not be surprised, provides an effective means of protection against parasites. The mucus produced by the body in just the right amount (if we are in balance) for the season provides our symbiotic bacteria a suitable place to live. Excessive mucus, on the other hand, creates a situation where the risk of harboring bad bacteria looms over us. When choosing foods from the spring grocery list, remember to eat as many of the leafy greens and root vegetables as possible to encourage intestinal health and balance of natural flora. To increase your children's consumption of leafy greens and roots, hide them in soups and stews. They are easily disguised, so your children will never know they had dandelions in their supper.

Preparing for Summer

The austere, low-fat foods of spring are important not only for their ability to clear out the accumulated fat and mucus that have built up over the winter, but also to prepare the body for summer. With the high sugar and carbohydrate content of the summer diet just around the corner, it is necessary to establish a baseline fat-burning metabolism in the spring. Eating the low-fat spring diet encourages the body to develop that baseline, providing a stable source of energy. This baseline allows the body to ingest the fruits of summer and utilize them effectively for energy. With this fat-burning foundation, the sugars of summer provide bursts of energy without creating the highs and lows of the blood sugar roller coaster ride.

During the long days and short nights of summer, the body requires an abundance of energy. This energy comes from the spring metabolism of winter's stored fat and the abundance of freshly harvested carbohydrates of summer.

The core of the body's energy metabolism comes from burning fat as fuel. This is one way that nature makes sure we never get on the blood sugar roller coaster in the first place. The spring months are the time of year when the energy centers are reset to burn fat so they are not destabilized by fluctuating blood sugar.

From One Season to the Next ...

We have not yet discussed the accumulation of a season's qualities as the season matures. Throughout each season, we see its properties build up and intensify. We have all noticed that the end of a long, cold, and dry winter is much more frigid; it is colder in February than in November. It is hotter in August and September than it is in June. Our bodies also feel these effects—thermal accumulation is the process by which our bodies build up heat throughout the summer months so that, just like the environment around us, at the end of the summer, our bodies are holding onto more heat.

The mechanism by which nature reduces the end-of-season accumulation is the climate change of the next season. Nature responds to the dryness of winter by flooding the environment and the body with moisture, warmth, and humidity in the spring. After the unending rain and mud of spring, nature provides the drying heat of summer to dry out the muddy earth. In our bodies, it helps to dry out any accumulated mucus left over from the spring.

We need to adjust our diets seasonally to go with the flow of these transitions, not against them. If we eat the standard American diet, high in mucus-producing foods, in the spring, and make no attempt to remove this springtime mucus, the heat of summer runs the risk of drying it into a hardened mucoid material. This dense, toxic junk can coat the intestinal wall and compromise assimilation and absorption of nutrients. It may take years for this to develop into a digestive problem, but it is a significant issue that can be completely avoided if we eat with nature's harvest.

Summer Refrigerants

The harvest of summer is rich in green vegetables and fruits, which are nature's way of cooling summer's accumulated heat. As the temperature rises throughout the summer, the harvest of more powerfully cooling foods increases.

If adequate amounts of cooling foods are not ingested during the hot summer months, this risk of becoming overheated increases. Although all kid-types experience the effects of accumulated

It is said that heat is the reason the leaves turn red in the fall. Accumulated summer heat rises to the trees' leaves, turning them beautiful reds and oranges. Ultimately they dry up and fall off. This same process happens in the body. You may have noticed that at the end of summer, the skin and sinuses are particularly dry and parched.

summer heat, summer kid-types are considerably more vulnerable to imbalances at this time of year. Their skin will be more susceptible to rashes, their sinuses to allergies and inflammation, and their tempers may flare. It is important for summer kid-types to be conscientious about eating cooling foods and avoiding spicy foods in the summer months, especially at the extremely hot end of the season.

An apple a day ... At the end of the summer, eating apples, drinking apple cider, making stewed apples and, of course, eating plenty of apple pies were all part of the traditional American life. Apples do two important things to help the body cope with the accumulated heat of summer. First, they are extremely cooling as a result of their sweet and astringent taste. Second, they are high in pectin and fiber, which clean out and detoxify the intestinal tract before the long winter rest.

If cooling and detoxifying measures are not taken, the body will move into winter carrying this dryness-causing heat. Even though the heat is mitigated by the cold of winter, the summer dryness in the body only continues to get worse as the further dryness of winter revs up.

The accumulated dryness irritates the mucous membranes, making them more reactive to pollens, pollutants, and respiratory irritants. These seasonal susceptibilities and patterns of imbalance can result in late summer allergies or hay fever (by definition, hay fever indicates an accumulation of heat or "fever" with associated respiratory symptoms). This imbalance can gain momentum as we move into cold and flu season. If the mucous membranes are not protected, they will continue to dry out even more, triggering the all-too-familiar reactive mucus that can breed viral and bacterial infections.

> To temper the intensity of the summer heat, nature offers us an abundance of apples, melons, pomegranates, and other sweet and cooling fruits.

Nature is doing its best to prevent this. It provides cooling fruits in the summer to prevent the heat from drying out the body. And in the winter season it provides a harvest of soothing and lubricating nuts, grains, oils, and meats—high-protein, high-fat foods that insulate and protect the mucous membranes.

 Parental Tip: If the heat of summer is countered with the cool summer harvest, and the accumulated dryness of winter is mitigated with the warm and insulating fall harvest, seasonal allergies and the ravages of colds and flus can become a distant memory.

Taste Counts

If all the grocery stores and supermarkets closed and we were forced to survive in the wilderness, we would eventually map out the good and bad sources of nutrition by tasting them. We would identify some herbs, roots, and leaves as nourishing; others we would learn to leave alone; still others we would find to have great therapeutic value. We would soon discover a science of natural nutrition based on how foods taste.

This science already exists, and this tasting and experimentation has already been done. It is one of the hallmarks of Ayurveda. Ayurveda classifies foods according to the "six tastes"—sweet, sour, salty, pungent, bitter, and astringent. The science of Ayurveda further categorizes foods by adding to the paired qualities of heavy/light, dry/oily, and hot/cold. This time-tested nutritional map, along with the knowledge of each individual kid-type and the associated seasons, provides the most comprehensive and natural means of nutrition available today.

In Sanskrit, the language of the Ayurvedic texts, the word for taste (*rasa*) also translates to mean emotion. The Ayurvedic texts state that each of the six tastes carries with it an emotional tone or quality. The tastes help to nurture and balance their corresponding emotional quality. For a meal to properly nourish the body, mind, and emotions—to be psycho-physiologically complete—it needs to include all six tastes.

I realize that getting children to appreciate even two of the six tastes can be a chore. But efforts to work with the tastes can have profound results. Simply by adjusting the tastes in the diet, an out-of-sorts child can be brought into line. By adding or removing a taste you can help restore a child to balance. You can work creatively to accomplish this by hiding these therapeutic tastes in your meals as spices, or in soups and stews.

The tastes can also offer a diagnostic tool for understanding your child's nutrition and imbalances. For example, if your child is complacent, he or she may be indulging in too much of the sweet taste; if your child is angry and beating up a younger sibling, then take away the salty chips.

Eighty Percent of Taste Is Actually Smell

The senses of taste and smell are intimately connected to each other and to the central workings of the brain. The sense of smell has direct access to the limbic system of the brain, which is the seat of our emotions. This is why smells can trigger memories or remembered feelings. Taste and smell are also directly wired to the hypothalamus, the master switchboard of the brain, which controls thirst and hunger and is responsible for neurochemical and hormonal regulation of the whole body. In short, the entire functioning of the body, mind, and emotions is modulated via the senses of smell and taste. The importance of these senses is unsurprising when we remember that they are the most ancient and primitive of our senses and that animals base their survival on the information they glean from them.

Now . . . How Can This Information Round Out a Parent's Nutritional Platform?

Sweet Taste

Sweet foods (except honey) increase spring and decrease summer and winter:

- Sugar, honey
- Rice
- Milk, cream, butter
- Wheat bread
- Meat

The sweet taste, when taken in its natural form (such as rice, bread, or pasta) provides a nutritional and emotional "satisfaction factor" to meals. Long-chain, slowly absorbed carbohydrates contain the sweet taste that provides us, and especially our nervous system, with energy. Without a taste of something sweet, it is common to leave the table unsatisfied, without being able to pinpoint exactly why.

Sweet taste balances the qualities of both winter and summer. It soothes and satisfies the nervous system (governed by winter in the body), and quickly feeds the impatient and hungry summer kid-type because it is absorbed into the bloodstream faster than any other food group. But too much sweet will increase spring properties, producing added weight, congestion, and eventually, lethargic behavior.

Sweet provides satisfaction that is not only physical, but also emotional. Sweet experiences and foods are those that are pleasant and comforting. On the other hand, too much sweet can over-stimulate the pleasure centers in the brain, leading to feelings of complacency, lethargy, or loss of motivation. Problems like obesity and compulsive eating disorders can also occur as a result of over-indulgence in the sweet taste. Sweet food (often in the form of junk food) is frequently abused in an attempt to make up for the lack of satisfaction in life. Sweets are then inappropriately tried and found guilty for causing a multitude of food and sugar addictions. As one part of a comprehensive approach for children with eating disorders, more attention should be placed on balancing the meals with all six tastes, as well as eating at the right time of day (as discussed in Chapter 6).

Sour Taste

Sour foods increase summer and spring and decrease winter:

- Lemon
- Cheese, yogurt
- Tomatoes, grapes, plums, sour fruits
- Wine

The experience of sour is quite the opposite of the calm, soothing nature of sweet. Sour is not warmly accepted by the body! Lemons, probably the thoroughbreds of the sour taste, are rarely eaten alone, but a little lemon juice provides a stimulating balance to a meal. Foods with primarily sour tastes are a little harder for the body to digest and stimulate an increase in heat—the body's digestive fire—in order to properly break them down. This stimulating heat is why we should have small amounts of sour in the diet.

Sour foods such as yogurt, cheeses, and sour fruits are usually qualitatively heavy, aggravating the already-heavy nature of the spring kid-type. They have a balancing effect on the light winter kid-types. Their heat-increasing properties tend to fire up the mental/emotional traits of summer kid-types, fueling their already aggressive and competitive nature.

The emotional effect of the sour taste is self-evident on the face of any child after sucking on his or her first lemon! The heat of the sour taste fires up our desire to accomplish goals and vanquish the opposition. This is a quality that is important to cultivate in a balanced manner. If the taste of sour is taken in excess, particularly by a summer kid-type, the usual enjoyment of competition can be "soured," leading to an unhealthy level of desire to overpower and vanquish the opposition, poor sportsmanship, and an increased likelihood of the child becoming a "sour-puss."

Salty Taste

Salty foods increase spring and summer, and decrease winter:

- Salt

Salt stimulates the digestive fire and is often used therapeutically when digestion is out of balance. This stimulating action is due in part to its heating effect. The heating nature of salt is easy to notice if you've ever gotten salt water in an open wound or in your eye and felt the stinging and burning of its heat. In the same way that salt melts snow or ice on the road, it also heats the body.

Pure summer kid-types should cut back on salt in the summer months, when heat is already accumulating. When taken in excess, salt can aggravate a summer kid-type, causing inflammatory skin disorders and intolerance to heat.

Salt Tablets

Salt, by its nature, attracts water. For decades, salt tablets were taken for any extensive activity in the heat. The rationale was that since we lose so much water through perspiration, salt replacement would safeguard the internal water supply, hence cooling the body and balancing electrolytes (minerals needed for muscle contraction). This theory is correct if we take just the right amount of salt. But what is the right amount? Multi-million dollar laboratories are still trying to determine the perfect balance of sugars and salts for best performance in the heat. But salt's properties of increasing heat are greater than the cooling properties derived from holding onto water. The net effect of taking in extra salt is usually to increase heat. Watch carefully how much salt you take in while exercising, especially in the heat of summer. Some salt is essential; too much can be overheating.

Emotionally, salt is like sour. It stimulates the driving, goal-oriented summer qualities of achievement. In excess, it can create unbalanced emotions of envy or resentment. Children with naturally aggressive minds may seek satisfaction from achievement of outward goals rather than from within. As a result, they don't enjoy themselves and become jealous of the accomplishments of others.

Bitter Taste

Bitter foods increase winter, and decrease summer and spring:

- Bitter greens (endive, romaine lettuce, collard greens)
- Spinach and other leafy greens
- Bitter cucumbers
- Tonic water
- Coffee
- Dark chocolate
- Turmeric, fenugreek

The taste of bitter is, in our society, probably the most ignored and neglected of the six tastes. The vegetable kingdom is spilling over with bitter tastes, yet, despite the fact that we have all heard the "eat your vegetables" refrain for as long as we can remember, 22% of Americans do not eat any vegetables. The American Heart and American Cancer Associations both recommend veggies for the prevention of disease and maintenance of good health. All of the leafy green vegetables, such as spinach, Swiss chard, romaine lettuce, arugula, and a variety of others, contain the bitter taste.

These light, bitter foods balance the heavy spring kid-types. They are cooling, which makes them good, especially for summer kid-types, to eat in the summer—just when nature provides them in abundance. The bitter and cooling plant aloe vera is well known for its healing properties in treating rashes, inflammations, and fever. Most bitter foods or spices have a similar therapeutic effect, but too much bitter can create excess lightness, aggravating the airy winter kid-types, who should eat less of them in the winter months.

Bitter is an important emotional quality included in a balanced diet to stabilize the pleasure of sweet. Too much pleasure without balance is said to have caused the downfall of the Roman Empire by creating a complacent and ultimately decadent society. Bitter allows sweet to bring satisfaction and pleasure without becoming addictive. But in excess, the bitter taste will ultimately overcome happy feelings, leaving one first bitter-sweet, and then just plain bitter.

Pungent Taste

Pungent foods increase summer and winter, and decrease spring:

- Cayenne and chili pepper
- Onions and garlic
- Radishes (including wasabi and horseradish)
- Ginger
- Mustard and mustard greens
- Spicy foods in general

Pungent is hot and spicy. Chili peppers, onions, and ginger are a few of the foods with a pungent taste. Their effect is to increase heat, experienced while eating (or even after eating!) a spicy Mexican meal. They help to stimulate and improve the digestive fire. This is why pungent foods are used as condiments or in cooking. Salsa with Mexican food, horseradish with meats, wasabi with sushi, and onions and garlic in Mediterranean food are common combinations.

Pungent foods should be used in moderation by summer kid-types, especially in the summer months. The increased heat of the summer environment, coupled with heat-increasing pungent foods, can send summer kid-types into imbalance, leading to rashes, heartburn, and ulcers. Fortunately, most kids naturally limit their intake of hot, spicy, pungent foods.

The pungent nature of spicy foods has a beneficial effect on breaking up the congestion and mucus often seen in respiratory conditions and spring kid-types. You may have experienced the effect a hot jalapeño pepper has in clearing your sinuses. These foods can be of immediate benefit to a spring kid-type experiencing a congestive bronchial condition or an asthmatic attack. Taken in moderation, pungent foods act to prevent the buildup of congestion.

Emotionally, pungent foods bring a spice, a bite, and a fire not only to digestion, but to the mind. But excess pungent tastes stoke the fires of summer kid-types, yielding quick tempers, irritability, aggressive behavior, and poor sportsmanship.

Astringent Taste

Astringent foods increase winter, and decrease summer and spring:

- Beans
- Lentils
- Apples, pears
- Cabbage, broccoli, cauliflower
- Potatoes
- Pomegranates

The astringent taste has a puckering and drying effect inside the mouth, and it is the least recognized taste in our society. Pomegranates are probably the most easily recognized astringent food. The astringent foods have a drying effect on the wet and congestive nature of spring, making these foods good for spring kid-types, particularly during the spring months.

Astringent foods are also cooling by nature. When you scan the list of astringent-dominated foods, consider when they are harvested—typically at the end of summer. These cooling foods: apples, pears, potatoes, and pomegranates, are ripe for eating at this time and help to dissipate excess heat.

Because of their light and drying effect, when eaten in excess, astringent foods will increase the properties of winter. The gas-producing qualities of astringent beans and lentils are an example of this. A winter kid-type complaining of constipation or experiencing abdominal gas should limit or avoid these dry and airy astringent foods, particularly in fall and winter.

Emotionally, the astringent taste is cooling and brings the mind and attention inward. Just the right amount of astringent can help balance spring and summer kid-types, keeping them energetic and cool, respectively. But in excess, the astringent taste will aggravate the nervous system triggering an overly withdrawn, shy, fearful, or phobic disposition, making it difficult to do justice to the natural abilities of your child.

The Six Ayurvedic Tastes:

Sweet	Sugar, milk, butter, rice, breads, pasta
Sour	Yogurt, lemon, cheese
Salty	Salt
Pungent	Spicy foods, ginger, hot peppers, cumin
Bitter	Green leafy vegetables, turmeric
Astringent	Beans, lentils, pomegranate

How the Six Tastes Affect the Winter, Summer, and Spring Kid-Types:

Decrease Winter	Sweet, Sour, Salty
Increase Winter	Pungent, Bitter, Astringent
Decrease Summer	Sweet, Bitter, Astringent
Increase Summer	Pungent, Sour, Salty
Decrease Spring	Pungent, Bitter, Astringent
Increase Spring	Sweet, Sour, Salty

The Six Qualities

Six Important Qualities to Keep in Mind When Considering the Effects of Food

Heavy and Light
Heavy—Wheat, beef, cheese
Light—Barley, chicken, skim milk

Oily and Dry:
Oily—Milk, soybeans, coconut
Dry—Honey, lentils, cabbage

Hot and Cold:
Hot—Pepper, honey, eggs
Cold—Mint, sugar, milk

Connecting the Six Tastes and the Six Qualities

Balances Winter	*Aggravates Winter*
Sweet—Heavy	Pungent—Light
Sour—Oily	Bitter—Dry
Salty—Hot	Astringent—Cold

Balances Summer	*Aggravates Summer*
Sweet—Cold	Pungent—Hot
Bitter—Heavy	Sour—Light
Astringent—Dry	Salty—Oily

Balances Spring	*Aggravates Spring*
Pungent—Light	Sweet—Heavy
Bitter—Dry	Sour—Oily
Astringent—Hot	Salty—Cold

Fruit

Fruits are made up predominantly of carbohydrates, vitamins, and minerals, with very little protein and fat. They are to be favored when they are in season, which for most fruits is the summer. They have a cooling influence, which is the antidote to the heat of summer. In the tropics, where heat is abundant year-round—fruits are harvested all year. Fruits are generally harvested when needed to compensate for environmental heat and to provide energy during the long days of the summer months.

In northern climates, there are no fruits naturally available in the winter. The nutritional call is for heavier foods to insulate and warm the body, protecting against the cold winter. Some fruits, however, that are grown in tropical areas, contain winter-balancing qualities of warmth, heaviness, and insulation-building fat. Avocados and bananas are two examples, and even though they are not harvested in Vermont in the winter, they are perfectly fine foods to eat during the cold months.

We tend to think of the avocado as a summer food, but its high fat content makes it a good winter fruit. It contains 25% fat, the fruit with the second highest fat content (after olives) in the world. In the avocado's native tropical areas, most varieties naturally mature for a fall and winter harvest. So nature again provides a food that gracefully remedies the cold and dry qualities of winter with its harvest of the avocado.

Many other fruits are okay in the winter because their sweet, sour, and heavy properties are an antidote to the dry, cold, and light qualities of winter. They can also be cooked to enhance their winter-balancing properties. For example, oranges, which are harvested in Florida in the early winter, contain qualities that balance winter—they are sweet, sour, and heavy, with a high water content. In areas where winters are mild, winter-harvested citrus fruits are a perfect antidote as the climate doesn't demand as many of the heavier winter remedies, like meat and nuts, that are needed in the north.

In the spring, most fruits are not yet ripe or ready to be harvested, so few fruits are recommended. Spring is, however, a perfect time for dry fruits. In farming communities, fruits would be dried in the fall, stored over the winter, and then eaten in the spring when the other harvest was sparse.

Fresh fruit juices concentrate the cooling effects of fruit, and can be difficult to digest. Spices like ginger, lemon juice, salt, cardamom, or clove can be added to enhance their digestibility. These spices provide a warming quality to the juice in the spring and winter.

Very sweet fruits like melons can be difficult to digest and can be spiced to enhance digestibility. Salt, lemon juice, and even chili pepper are used on melons throughout the world to enhance taste and improve digestibility. However, melons don't mix well with other foods and are best taken alone. Sour fruits like lemon, pineapple, papaya, and cranberries are easy to digest and can be eaten with other foods. Most fruits mix well with grains but not with vegetables.

Vegetables

Many of the vegetables that are the mainstays of our current diet are harvested in the spring and summer. But the American diet used to consist of more root vegetables than it does now. These root veggies are typically harvested in both the spring and fall. In the fall they are harvested to be eaten as warm, nourishing foods; in the winter and spring they are harvested to be anti-mucus, low-fat antidotes to the heavy, wet months.

In Europe, root vegetables like parsnips, turnips, beets, and fennel are still a significant part of fall and spring diets.

Most of the heavy, warming root veggies like beets, carrots, and potatoes are harvested in the fall. They store well and are eaten throughout the winter and spring. These foods are full of vitamins and minerals, and their high-quality nutrition is great to combat the light and dry qualities of winter.

The vegetables that are the first harvest of the spring—spinach, kale, Swiss chard, and mustard greens—all to stimulate cleansing in the deep tissues as the body transitions from winter to spring. Adding spices (pepper, salt, mustard seed, cumin, coriander, or asafoetida) to leafy greens while cooking enhances their digestibility.

Pungent vegetables like onions and chilies also help burn off the excess fat and protein that was stored in the winter; these keep well over the winter to be eaten in the spring. Also, many of the natural diuretic veggies remove excess water that the body tends to hold onto in the spring. Nature provides an antidote to spring's heavy qualities in the form of the spring-harvested vegetables including: parsley, cilantro, lettuce, watercress, and asparagus. Others, like broccoli, potatoes, carrots, and celery, although they are not harvested in the spring, have useful spring-antidote qualities.

With the harvest of cucumbers, zucchini, okra, peas, and celery, the qualities of the summer veggies shift from being cleansing and fat-free to being more nutritious and cooling. These vegetables provide us with nutrition and energy to endure the long, demanding days of summer. They are harmonious with the beginning of the summer fruit harvest, which is dedicated to both cooling and providing a rich source of energy.

COOKING TIPS:

Raw vegetables are good in the summer.
Cooked vegetables are good in the winter.
Salads are good in the spring.
Pickled foods are good in the winter.
Cooking with oil is good in the winter.
Salted foods are good in the winter.
Spiced foods are good in the winter and spring.
Deep-frying is not recommended for summer or spring.

Grains

Grains are harvested in the fall to provide us with a high-protein, high-fat, and adequate-carbohydrate source to eat in the winter. Grains store well and last throughout the year, so they can be eaten in moderation anytime, and they blend well with other foods.

Grains are predominantly heavy, making them a good food to balance a winter kid-type and a good food to combat the dry, cold winter. Some types of grain are heavier than others and are better in the winter, while some are less heavy making them appropriate in the spring and summer. Some, like barley, rye, buckwheat, and corn, are especially good in the spring due to their water-removing diuretic properties. The high-protein warming, building grains that are better in the winter include: wheat, oats, brown and white rice, quinoa, and amaranth. Dried grains like granola are better in the wet spring and not as good in the dry winter.

Because yeast produces gas, which is what makes bread rise, yeast breads can be more difficult to digest in the winter. Toasting helps improve digestibility; but yeasted breads are better eaten in the summer when the heat is high and digestion is strong.

Legumes

Legumes are the fall-harvested beans such as lentils, black beans, and kidney beans, and should not be confused with the spring-harvested green or string beans. Legumes can cause the body to produce gas due to the hard fiber shell that protects the bean from rot and rancidity. The benefit of this shell is that beans are able to last for years if needed. Although we may think of beans as a good winter food since they are harvested in the fall, they are actually more appropriate in the spring and summer when their gassy properties are less problematic than in the already-airy winter.

> Mung beans, preferably split yellow mung dal, and tofu are two of the easiest beans to eat in the airy winter.

Beans can be eaten in the winter and make a good protein and nutrient source as long as they are not eaten excessively and they are sprouted, soaked, parboiled, and/or well spiced. Sprouting any type of bean makes it more nutritious as sprouting increases the bean's chlorophyll content. It also improves digestibility since the fibrous shell is broken when beans sprout. Soaking and parboiling beans improves digestibility by reducing their gas-producing qualities.

> Helpful spices for cooking with beans are: onions, hing (asafoetida), cumin, fennel, cayenne, salt, pepper, cardamom, or epazote (Mexican tea).

Nuts and Seeds

Fall-harvested nuts and seeds are loaded with fat and protein, making them the perfect food for the winter season. Because nuts are heavy, they can sometimes be hard to digest; soaking them overnight or peeling their skins (especially with almonds) makes them easier to digest. Nut milks provide an easily assimilated source of nutrients, but nut butters are hard to digest. Eat nut butters in small quantities and add spices to increase digestibility.

> Soaked and peeled almonds are one of the best protein sources available.

Roasting Nuts:

Unroasted nuts are good in spring and summer (moderate amounts in the summer).

Lightly roasted nuts are good in the winter.

Dry-roasted nuts are best in the spring in small amounts and not recommended in the winter.

Honey-roasted nuts are not recommended because of the cooked honey (details in Chapter 3).

Dairy

Although dairy products have been give a very bad rap from the natural health community, there is some cream to skim off the top of this subject. First, let's look at the way most Americans consume dairy products. The two most common forms of dairy products consumed in the U.S. are cold milk on cereal and ice cream. In traditional dairy-herding cultures in Europe, Africa, India (and not that long ago in America), milk was rarely used cold. The milk was taken from cow to table (after boiling) and consumed warm. The cows it came from were antibiotic-, pesticide-, and hormone-free.

We, on the other hand, drink milk from cows that have been injected with growth hormones and antibiotics and have eaten a diet loaded with pesticides. We pasteurize the milk to kill anything that the antibiotics haven't, and then, to increase its shelf-life, we blast it through a tiny filter with extremely high pressure during the process of homogenization.

When we compare traditional milk-drinking practices to the modern American ones, it is just not the same. I agree with the dairy critics that the best way to give your child a cold in the winter or spring is to feed them cold cow's milk on their cereal, or milkshakes with dinner. When milk and dairy products are consumed cold, the mucus-producing qualities in milk are dramatically increased.

Pasteurized and homogenized milk is, in my opinion, very difficult to digest and contributes to why so many people today are lactose-intolerant. Before milk was so highly processed and when it was used in a more traditional style—raw, warm, and additive-free— people had fewer problems digesting it and everyone seemed quite fine. It was only after homogenization came on the scene in the 1950s and '60s that milk started getting a bad name. Lactose intolerance increased and cholesterol levels and obesity in America started to rise to the all-time high we see today.

It can be difficult to find good whole milk to drink that has not been homogenized. But, there is good milk available in almost all the states that allow the sale of non-homogenized milk. Homogenization is a process done purely for convenience, with no health benefit. In fact, it's detrimental because it drastically changes the qualities of the milk. In Ayurvedic medicine, it is believed that the homogenization process makes the fat in milk indigestible by breaking down important digestive enzymes that naturally occur in whole, raw milk. The indigestibility of the milk causes the accumulation of toxins, or *ama,* in the bloodstream when used as a food.

In Western medicine, it is understood that the homogenization process allows the dangerous enzyme xanthine oxidase in the milk to enter the bloodstream instead of being excreted from the body. In the heart and circulatory system, this enzyme damages the membranes of the lining of the heart and the blood vessels, allowing cholesterol to accumulate and deposit in the arteries and the heart. In my opinion, homogenization of milk is to blame for making milk indigestible.

If you choose to buy non-homogenized milk, it is often labeled as "cream-top" milk because the cream separates from the rest of the milk when the particles are not forced through the filter.

> It was never traditional to drink milk in a large glass, ice-cold, all at once. Milk was usually used in cooking, warm on hot cereal, or as a cup of hot milk.

Pasteurization changes the milk from its natural state by heating it to kill any infective microorganisms. Before hygienic practices were as stringent as they are today, this practice saved many lives by making milk safe to be sold in the marketplace. In many states, it is not legal to buy raw milk in a store for sanitary reasons, but it can be obtained in many areas. If you intend to buy raw milk, get to know a farm and its hygiene practices. The milk should also be quickly boiled and then allowed to cool at home before drinking. This will destroy harmful bacteria while retaining most of the valuable nutrients, and make it easier for your body to digest.

Pasteurization does not have the same negative health implications as homogenization. If you cannot buy raw milk fresh from a farm, try to find pasteurized, non-homogenized milk. The process of pasteurization takes place below boiling temperature, so it does not completely break down the milk's protein chains, which is why you need to boil raw milk. The incomplete process of protein breakdown makes the milk more difficult to digest, according to Paul Pitchford, author of *Healing With Whole Foods*.

Human milk contains four times as much water-soluble whey protein as cow's milk and half as much casein. While whey is easy for us to digest, casein is more difficult, which may be why, in Ayurvedic medicine, the milk was always brought to a quick boil before use. Goat milk, on the other hand, does not need to be brought to a boil to increase its digestibility.

Warm milk:

We have all heard of the folk remedy of a warm glass of milk before bed to make you feel or sleep better. It is still common in traditional cultures to have warm milk at night, and it is often recommended in Ayurveda. Spice the milk with ginger, cardamom, cinnamon, mustard seed, cayenne, cumin, nutmeg, or honey for flavor variations.

Adding spices to milk helps balance its mucus-producing properties. If finding non-homogenized milk is difficult, but you or your children want to continue drinking milk, spice it and take it warm

> Milk does not combine well with other foods; doing so can cause digestive problems.

or hot. Try not to use cold milk in the morning when digestion is at its slowest.

In some cultures warm spiced raw milk is given to children for head colds—completely opposite to modern Western and natural approaches to head-cold management. But if the cold is caused by the excessive dryness in the sinuses, which is all-too-common in winter's cold and flu season, then the use of milk with warming pungent spices can open blocked sinuses. And the hot milk itself has a demulcent or lubricating effect to combat the dryness of winter. I don't use this recipe much for my children or patients—I prefer to use herbs to accomplish the same thing without the risk of contributing to further mucus production.

If there were one season to avoid milk it would be the wet spring. During this time of year, cold milk will increase mucus production and precipitate a cold or infection. Drink milk in moderation in the winter—and not first thing in the morning or in the evening with other foods. Hot spiced milk before bed is not a problem. The best time of year to enjoy milk is the summer when the cooling qualities of milk are a natural antidote to the heat.

Realistically, finding healthy non-pasteurized and non-homogenized milk is difficult. Many parents have found it easier to just stop feeding their children milk. There are many substitutes on the market today such as rice milk, soy milk, and almond and nut milks, all of which kids typically can acquire a taste for. In our house, we drink primarily Rice Dream on cereal and offer cow's milk to the children with their cereal as a treat. We will do this more often in the summer than in the spring, fall, or winter.

It may not always be possible to restrict your child's intake of milk products during the cold seasons, in which case I suggest using trikatu, which is effective for breaking down hard-to-digest foods.

Trikatu and Dairy

I introduced trikatu in Chapter 4 as the herbal formula to be used on pizza-delivery nights. It can also be used on any occasion before a meal to help break down hard-to-digest foods. For kids, cold milk on cereal is one of those. Taking trikatu is an extremely effective way to offset the mucus-producing and cold-causing properties of milk products. One capsule or 1/2 to 1 teaspoon of the herbal honey paste (equal parts herb and honey) taken be taken either before or after the meal.

Meat

If you lived in Vermont, Colorado, Alaska, or Montana 100 years ago, you would having eaten meat in the winter or died. That was just the way it was. Now it seems somewhat decadent to be killing animals in the summer while apples are rotting on the grass because we choose to eat meat rather than fill up on the foods nature has provided for us in abundance. In the summer, the natural tendency is to eat less meat and consume more seasonal fruits and veggies. Come winter, when it's cold and dry, meat is a perfect antidote to the severity of the season.

Protein helps build the body, which is why bodybuilders live on protein powders and amino acids to pump them up. In the winter, the body is actively storing fat, protein, minerals, and vitamins. If we do not provide those nutrients in the winter our body will be unsatisfied and will crave inappropriate foods all year long. Meat is a winter food that helps the body store these nutrients.

Many vegetarians find themselves protein-deficient in the winter because of the high protein requirements of the body at this time of year. In our society, it is difficult to be a healthy vegetarian because high-quality vegetarian meals can be hard to get in restaurants, and cooking such meals is time-consuming. To have a healthy vegetarian family, parents would have to cook at least two hours a day to provide the family with the proper amount of vegetarian nutrition. With everyone being so busy in this day and age, it is rare to find that kind of time. Although I truly believe that a vegetarian diet is the most healthful diet for human beings, in our culture it is extremely difficult, if not impossible, to maintain.

Because of this, I don't recommend a vegetarian diet for children.

Many vegetarian kids and adults do not maintain a high-enough quality diet; they then become addicted to sugar for their nutritional energy instead of obtaining energy from a well-balanced vegetarian diet. They often complain of hypoglycemia and energy highs and lows as a result of riding the blood sugar roller coaster.

 Parental Tip: Children who insist on being vegetarians need to be supported by an effort to feed them protein in the form of nuts, seeds, whole grains, soy products, beans and legumes, dairy, and even whey-based protein shakes. Whey is the easiest-to-digest protein source for kids' shakes because it is water soluble. Soy protein, like most bean protein, is heavy and hard to break down, particularly for the delicate digestive system of a child.

Decoding the Grocery Store

The shelves at the supermarket are laden with foods whose seasonal attributes we may be unfamiliar with. The 3-Season Diet Grocery List at the end of the chapter includes foods from around the world. The three-season diet uses a global approach. Foods harvested in each season are listed so eating will not be a restrictive or austere experience. In fact, many families do not even realize the transition to the three-season plan. These foods are typically what the family already enjoys, often crave, and before long, prefer.

By using this grocery list, everyone in the home eats the same food, which makes shopping and meal preparation pain-free. Obtaining the medicinal benefits of foods when they are in season is a profound dietary practice that can have a significant influence on your health.

Generally, eat a winter diet in the winter months from November through February. Eat a spring diet from March through June and a summer diet from July through October. Remember that there is a graceful transition between seasons that will vary from location to location geographically.

Transitioning from Season to Season

We experience the seasonal transitions when, at the end of winter, spring starts to peek its head in and out, alternating warm 60-degree days with snowy ones; when the rains of spring start to trickle away; or when the sharp cold-snaps of autumn mix with the summer sun. During these times, you can select foods from both lists. Eat spinach at lunch from the spring list on a warm day when the sun appears and then eat a hearty soup off the winter list if the weather gets cold that evening. For each of the seasonal transitions, choose foods that favor the qualities of the weather that day, or the climate that appears during that meal. Following this rule will make applying the dietary changes as smooth and graceful as the seasonal change itself.

When to Follow a Body-Type Diet?

Some body-type-related conditions would be helped by under-standing how to modify a seasonal diet according to the kid-type. For a child with an extreme kid-type, modify the diet by starting the season-appropriate diet early and sticking with it. This is not a usual adjustment, generally speaking, but it may come in handy.

For medical reasons and for the treatment of certain imbal-ances it is common to recommend a specific winter, summer, or spring diet outside its respective season. Usually, this is used for only short periods of time to help bring the body back into balance and not as a permanent diet. If our diets do not change with the seasons, it will be only a matter of time before the body begins to crave the missing foods of nature's harvest.

How To Use the Grocery List

In the appropriate season, circle all the foods on that list that you like. Eat as much and as many of those foods as you like while using common sense. Foods from the other lists can be eaten—just be sure to eat a substantial amount of the in-season foods. Avoid foods which are known triggers for individual symptoms until the body starts to naturally reset its balance.

The 3-Season Grocery List

Many foods are havested in two or more seasons.

An asterisk (*) indicates the best food for that season.

WINTER	SUMMER	SPRING
FRUIT		
Apples (cooked)	Apples*	Apples
Apricots	Apricots*	
Bananas*	Bananas	
	Cranberries*	Cranberries
Cherries	Cherries (ripe)*	
Coconuts (ripe)*	Coconuts (green or ripe)*	
Dates	Dates	
		Dried Fruit (all)
Figs*	Figs	
Grapes*	Grapes*	
Grapefruit*		Grapefruit
Guavas	Guavas*	
Lemons (improve digestion)*		
Limes*		
Mangos*	Mangos*	
	Melons (all)*	
Cantaloupe	Cantaloupe*	
Oranges*	Oranges (sweet)	
Papaya*	Papaya (small amounts)	Papaya
Peaches (skin can heat in excess)	Peaches (ripe or peeled)*	
Nectarines	Nectarines	
Pears (ripe)	Pears*	Pears
Pineapples	Pineapples (sweet)*	
Persimmons*	Persimmons*	
Plums	Plums (ripe)*	
Pomegranates (sweet)	Pomegranates*	Pomegranates (sour)
	Raspberries	Raspberries
	Blackberries*	Blackberries
	Blueberries*	Blueberries
Strawberries	Strawberries	Strawberries
Tangerines*	Tangerines (sweet)	

WINTER	SUMMER	SPRING
VEGETABLES		
	Alfalfa Sprouts*	Alfalfa Sprouts*
Artichoke Hearts	Artichokes*	Artichokes
	Asparagus*	Asparagus*
Avocados	Avocados (in moderation)	
	Green Beans	Green Beans*
	Mung Bean Sprouts	Mung Bean Sprouts*
Beets*		
	Bell Peppers*	Bell Peppers
	Bitter Melons*	Bitter Melons
	Broccoli*	Broccoli
Brussels Sprouts*		Brussels Sprouts*
	Cabbage*	Cabbage*
Carrots*		Carrots*
	Cauliflower*	Cauliflower*
	Celery*	Celery*
	Chicory	Chicory*
Chilies*		Chilies (dried)
	Cilantro*	Cilantro
	Dandelions*	Dandelions
Hot Peppers		Hot Peppers*
Corn	Corn	Corn*
	Cucumbers*	
	Eggplant*	
Garlic*		Garlic*
Ginger		Ginger*
	Hibiscus*	Hibiscus
Jerusalem Artichokes	Jerusalem Artichokes*	
	Kale*	Kale*
	Lettuce*	Lettuce*
	Mushrooms	Mushrooms*
	Mustard Greens	Mustard Greens*
Okra	Okra*	
Onions		Onions*
Parsley*	Parsley*	Parsley*
	Peas	Peas*

WINTER	SUMMER	SPRING
VEGETABLES CONTINUED		
	Snow Peas	
Potatoes (mashed or steamed)	Potatoes*	Potatoes (baked)*
Pumpkin*	Pumpkin	
Seaweed (cooked)*	Seaweed*	Seaweed*
	Spinach (not in excess)	Spinach*
	Swiss Chard (not in excess)	Swiss Chard*
Acorn Squash	Acorn Squash*	
Winter Squash*	Winter Squash	
	Zucchini*	
	Radishes (in moderation)	Radishes*
Tomatoes*	Tomatoes (sweet)	
Sweet Potatoes*	Sweet Potatoes (in moderation)	
	Turnips	Turnips*
	Watercress*	Watercress*

WINTER	SUMMER	SPRING
NUTS/SEEDS		
Almonds*		
Brazil Nuts*		
Cashews*		
Coconuts	Coconuts*	
Filbert Nuts*		Filbert Nuts (in moderation)
Macadamias*	Macadamias	
Flax Seed*		Flax Seed
Pecans*		
Peanuts (raw)		
Walnuts*		
	Lotus Seeds*	
Pinyon Seeds*	Pinyon Seeds	Pinyon Seeds
Pistachios*		
	Pumpkin Seeds*	Pumpkin Seeds
Sunflower Seeds	Sunflower Seeds*	Sunflower Seeds

WINTER	SUMMER	SPRING
LEGUMES		
		All Sprouted Beans*
	Aduki*	Aduki
	Black Gram*	Black Gram
	Garbanzo*	Garbanzo
	Fava*	Fava
	Goya	Goya*
	Kidney	Kidney*
		Lentils*
	Lima	Lima*
Mung Beans*	Mung Beans*	Mung Beans*
Tofu	Tofu*	
	Split Pea*	Split Pea*

WINTER	SUMMER	SPRING
GRAINS		
Amaranth*		
Barley (in moderation)		Barley*
Buckwheat (in moderation)		Buckwheat*
Corn (in moderation)		Corn*
Millet (in moderation)		
Oats*		
Rice		
Brown Rice*		
Quinoa*		
Rye (in moderation)		Rye*
Spelt		
Wheat*	Wheat	

WINTER	SUMMER	SPRING
CONDIMENTS		
Carob	Carob	Carob
Chocolate*		Chocolate
Mayonnaise		
Salt		
Vinegar		
Pickles		

WINTER	SUMMER	SPRING
DAIRY		
Butter*	Butter*	
Buttermilk*		
Cheese*	Cheese (in moderation)	
Cottage Cheese*	Cottage Cheese	
Cream*	Cream*	
Ghee*	Ghee*	Ghee (in moderation)
	Ice Cream*	
Kefir*		
Milk (low-fat, not cold)	Milk*	Milk (skim or avoid)
Sour Cream*		
Yogurt (plain)*	Yogurt (sweet)	Yogurt (low-fat, in moderation)

WINTER	SUMMER	SPRING
MEAT & FISH		
Beef*		
Chicken*	Chicken (in moderation)	Chicken (in moderation)
Duck*		
Lamb*		
Lobster*		
Pork*	Pork	
Turkey*	Turkey	Turkey
Venison*		
Ocean Fish*		
Freshwater Fish	Freshwater Fish	Freshwater Fish
Crab*		
Oysters*		
Shrimp*		
Eggs*	Eggs (in moderation)	Eggs (in moderation)

WINTER	SUMMER	SPRING
SWEETENERS		
Raw Sugar	Raw Sugar	
Honey		Honey*
Molasses		
Rice Syrup	Rice Syrup	
Maple Syrup		

WINTER	SUMMER	SPRING
OILS		
Almond*		
Avocado*	Avocado (in moderation)	
	Canola	Canola
Castor*		
		Corn*
Coconut*	Coconut*	
Flax*		Flax
Mustard*		Mustard
Olive*	Olive*	
Peanut*		
Safflower*		Safflower*
Sesame*		
	Soy*	Soy
Sunflower	Sunflower	Sunflower

WINTER	SUMMER	SPRING
BEVERAGES		
Alcohol		
		Coffee
		Black Tea
		Sparkling Water
	Herbal Tea	
Ginger*		Ginger*
Cinnamon		Cinnamon
Cloves		Cloves
Cardamom		Cardamom
Orange Peel		Orange Peel
Chamomile	Chamomile	
Mint	Mint	
	Alfalfa	Alfalfa
	Dandelion*	Dandelion*
	Chicory	Chicory
	Strawberry Leaf	Strawberry Leaf
	Hibiscus	Hibiscus

WINTER	SUMMER	SPRING
SPICES		
Anise	Anise	Anise
Asafoetida (Hing)		Asafoetida (Hing)
Basil		Basil
Bay Leaf		Bay Leaf
Black Pepper		Black Pepper
Chamomile	Chamomile	Chamomile
Caraway		Caraway
Cardamom		Cardamom
Cayenne		Cayenne
Cinnamon		Cinnamon
Clove		Clove
Coriander	Coriander*	Coriander
Cumin	Cumin (in moderation)	Cumin
Dill		Dill
Fennel	Fennel	Fennel
Fenugreek		Fenugreek
Garlic		Garlic
Ginger	Ginger (in moderation)	Ginger
Horseradish		Horseradish
Marjoram		Marjoram
Mustard		Mustard
Nutmeg		Nutmeg
Oregano		Oregano
Peppermint	Peppermint	Peppermint
Poppy Seeds		Poppy Seeds
Rosemary	Rosemary (in moderation)	Rosemary
Saffron	Saffron	Saffron
Sage		Sage
Spearmint	Spearmint	Spearmint
Thyme		Thyme
Turmeric	Turmeric	Turmeric

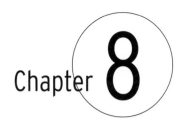

Chapter 8

Secret 7—Is Your Home Chemical-
and Allergen-Free?

The Environmental Protection Agency (EPA), as part of the 1989 Indoor Air Quality Act, reported that levels of indoor air pollutants were three to seven times higher than levels measured outdoors. In the same study, the EPA reported that toxic chemicals found in the home are three times more likely to cause cancer than outdoor airborne pollutants. What is surprising is that this toxicity did not come from the weed-killers in the garage, but the household cleaners and personal-care products found in your kitchen and bathroom! In 1989, The National Institute for Occupational Safety and Health analyzed 2,983 chemical ingredients in personal-care products and found 884 that were toxic and potentially harmful. Many of these chemicals are linked to allergies, breathing difficulties, and colds because they irritate the airways and trigger excessive mucus production.

These chemicals don't just cause colds, or irritate the mucus membranes—they can be fatal. Every year between 5 and 10 million reported poisonings are caused by the ingestion of common products found in almost every home. According to a 1999 report published in the *American Journal of Emergency Medicine*, 53% of these poisonings involve children under the age of 6. Items listed as creating a high risk for poisoning in children are household chemicals, plants, prescription drugs, and cosmetics, all commonly found in most American homes. They may be items we don't think of as being dangerous. For example, easily accessible liquid dish soap is the leading cause of poisonings in the home for children under the age of 6, adding up to 2.1 million accidental poisonings per year. This may be due to the fact that most brands of liquid soap contain formaldehyde and ammonia, both of which are on the toxic ingredients list that appears later in this chapter. It's surprising and distressing to learn that common products we use every day contain deadly ingredients. Ridding your home of these products is the first step toward a safer, healthier home.

Poisoning is not the only danger; household chemicals have also been linked to other serious conditions. In one 15-year EPA study, women who worked in the home had a 54% higher rate of death from cancer than women who worked outside the home. This study concluded that the increased death rate was due to daily exposure to the airborne toxins from hazardous chemicals found in ordinary household products. Women who work at home are not the only people who are vulnerable to this exposure. According to the EPA, there are three groups of people primarily affected by indoor air pollution—infants and toddlers, the elderly, and the chronically ill—because they spend more time indoors and their immune systems are weaker.

Children are clearly bearing the brunt of our chemical irresponsibility. Diseases that used to only develop later in life are now appearing in people at younger ages, and diseases that once were rare are now occurring more frequently. In 1901, cancer occurred in 1 out of every 8,000 people. The current cancer rate has risen to 1 in 3 people and, according to the American Cancer Society, will soon rise to 1 in 2. Cancer is the number-two killer of children—second only to accidental poisonings. According to the National Cancer Institute, the rate of cancer among American children has risen nearly 1% per year since 1977.

While the exact cause for this increase in cancer is still unknown, chemical toxicity is high on the list of suspects. The Consumer Protection Agency found that 150 chemicals commonly used in American homes are connected to allergies, birth defects, cancer, and psychological disorders. Just by reducing—not even eliminating—the carcinogens from our home environments, we would save at least 50,000 lives a year now taken by cancer, according to Dr. Lee Davis, the former adviser to the Secretary of Health.

> There is no question that the quality of the air we breathe and the water we drink, particularly for children, has a significant impact on our health.

Kids today catch more colds, suffer more from asthma, take more Ritalin, have more allergies, and are generally less healthy than kids were 20 to 30 years ago. The cause, I am sure, is a combination of many factors, including environmental toxicity. I attempt to discuss most of these in this in the upcoming chapters.

The high levels of toxic chemicals in the air and water are a recent phenomenon. Although we may think that the government monitors the plethora of chemicals sold and used, we cannot assume that the products we buy and the water we drink have been completely and scientifically evaluated for their long-term health risks. The Consumer Product Safety Commission (CPSC) was created to protect us, but it is not adequately funded or staffed to effectively evaluate the vast numbers of toxic products on the market. Even, if it did find a toxic product, the under-funded CPSC is likely not strong enough to battle the lobbying efforts of the Chemical Specialties Manufacturers Association, which represents the multi-billion dollar soap and detergent industry.

Not only are products inadequately tested, but the United States Code of Federal Regulations exempts manufacturers from full labeling of products if they are used for personal, family, or household care. Poison-control experts cannot rely on product labels to effectively and safely treat accidental poisonings because they are often incomplete or even missing.

Currently, there are approximately 72,000 chemicals legally registered with the EPA as ingredients in cleaning products, most of which have been introduced since 1950. The federal government has banned a small list of less than 100 chemicals that are too toxic to be used in cleaning products. Less than 10% of these registered chemicals have been completely studied and evaluated for their impact on human health and the environment.

According to Herbert Needleman, M.D., in his book, *Raising Children Toxic Free,* "We are by default conducting a massive clinical toxicology trial, and our children are the experimental animals." He goes on to say, "Developing cells in children's bodies are more susceptible to damage than adult cells that have completed development, especially for the central nervous system. During the development of a child from conception through adolescence, there are particular windows most vulnerable to environmental hazards. Most disturbing, until a child is approximately 13 months of age, they have virtually no ability to fight the biological and neurological effects of toxic chemicals."

Unfortunately, the manufacture and sale of cleaning and personal-care products is big business, and in our world of capitalism and consumerism we cannot assume, particularly as parents, that manufacturers have taken the proper precautions to ensure that a product is safe to use.

I encourage replacing popular brands of detergents and bleaches with natural products that are good for your health, your family, and the environment. Later in the chapter, I take you step-by-step through freeing your home of the many common allergens that can be directly linked to your children's colds or asthma. First I want to tell a story about how the information I've shared so far saved my son's life.

Treating our children is not as simple as giving an antibiotic for a cold or an inhaler for a wheeze. Understanding how children's excessive mucus production can weaken their immunity, understanding their individual natures while keeping close tabs on their digestive integrity, maintaining adequate hydration, feeding them foods at the appropriate time of day in line with the season, knowing their kid-types, and maintaining a home environment that is toxin-free, all play important roles in keeping your family healthy.

Secret Seven: The seventh heath secret is to keep your home environment free of toxic products. Major factors in our mental, physical and emotional health may be the air we breathe inside our own homes, our sheets and pillow cases, the clothes we wear, the perfumes we buy and the cleaners we use. By reducing the toxic chemicals in your home, you can improve the health of your family.

My 9-Month-Old Professor

When my fifth child, Jensen, was 9 months old, all of the health factors I stress throughout this book came into play—but the most significant one was the impact of chronic and cumulative exposure to chemicals in common household products. This exposure nearly cost him his life.

The Fine Line Between Life and Death

When infants are cutting their teeth it is common for them to drool more and for their noses to run a lot. Jensen was no exception: he drooled continuously and had a runny nose between the ages of 6 and 11 months. He had a tough time breaking in his teeth; he drooled and dripped like no other and then soon developed a cough. But he never once came down with a fever, stopped smiling, became cranky, or appeared to be sick, other than his nagging, persistent cough. His incessant teething was causing him to make so much mucus that he had a hard time shaking the cough. His nose ran with the clear mucus typical of a teething baby. Luckily, the mucus never became yellow, which can indicate an infection, and his mood and energy were always good.

We all thought that even though he was coughing, he would be fine once his teeth came in. Unfortunately, this wasn't the case, but here's where it got tricky. His cough stopped, his nose just about stopped running, and Jensen seemed pretty much back to normal; his eating, energy, and sleep were all good. Two healthy weeks passed and then right after the house had been cleaned one afternoon, Jensen started wheezing, just a little. It persisted into that evening and by eight o'clock that night it was clear this little guy needed help breathing.

We raced Jensen to the emergency room where he was given Albuterol and oxygen to clear his airway and help his breathing. Albuterol is a commonly prescribed bronchodilator for kids. In the emergency room, they took X-rays, listened to Jensen's lungs, and then told us his lungs were clear but that he probably had a reactive airway. This meant that he had had an allergic asthmatic attack, possibly due to the cleaning products used in the house. We brought some of the Albuterol treatments home and he started to improve.

The next day we took Jensen to our pediatrician's office where our nurse practitioner, Pat Frazier, saw him. After she listened to his lungs, she reported that they were definitely *not* clear. We told her the results from his X-rays and exam at the emergency room the night before; the doctor at the E.R. had said that his X-rays were normal and his lungs were clear. Pat disagreed, "I am sure they are not clear. I think he has pneumonia." She immediately called the hospital and spoke with the radiologist who was at that time reviewing the previous night's X-rays. He agreed with Pat's assessment that Jensen had been misdiagnosed.

The emergency room doctor had misread both Jensen's X-rays and his lung sounds. Jensen had bilateral pneumonia but was treated with Albuterol for an allergic reaction. Hearing this more serious diagnosis was scary. When we took Jensen in to the emergency room, he did not have a fever, there had been no cough for the past two weeks, and he showed no other noticeable symptoms, so this was not only a frightening diagnosis, but a perplexing one.

Obviously the emergency room doctor misread the X-rays. He was probably just not used to listening to infant lung sounds and missed the congestion. Unfortunately, his mistake could have cost

Jensen's life. This was only the first of many lessons we learned from this experience: make sure your doctor is an expert at listening to lung and breathing sounds with a stethoscope. I was so impressed with how carefully and accurately Pat listened to Jensen's lungs. There was no doubt in her mind that his lungs were congested, but her perceptive diagnosis of pneumonia still came as a surprise.

In all my years of practice working with health-care practitioners, Pat was the first one who really took the time and had the skill to hear everything in my child's lungs. Her diagnosis was life-saving. This type of listening skill is important not only for critical cases, like Jensen's, but for less severe cases as well. A doctor who is a confident auscultator of lung sounds will be less likely to prescribe antibiotics unnecessarily. A doctor who does not possess that skill and is in doubt about what he or she hears will be more likely to recommend antibiotics just to be on the safe side.

This makes more homework for us parents. Be very alert and watch your doctor carefully as he or she listens to your child's lungs. If the doctor gives only a brief and cursory listen to your child's lungs, or if you have a baby who is fussing or crying and you have a sense that the doctor did not hear every part of the lung clearly, and this same doctor routinely prescribes antibiotics, it might be time to find a doctor with better diagnostic skills.

Lesson One: Be sure your doctor is an expert at listening to your child's lungs. When you find a master, you will be amazed at how much he or she can tell you about your child's respiratory health and the seriousness of the condition in question.

For Jensen's new diagnosis of pneumonia, he was given a course of antibiotics along with the home Albuterol treatments to keep his lungs open. He bounced right back on this regimen. But a second life-threatening mistake was made at this point, this time by the pharmacy who gave us only a five-day course of antibiotics instead of the prescribed ten. Five days of antibiotics were not nearly enough to knock out bilateral pneumonia. This small error at the pharmacy once again almost cost Jensen his life. It is amazing how aware parents have to be and how easy it is to make mistakes.

On the eighth day Jensen had a relapse. We were eating lunch at a restaurant where, that day, a busboy sprayed window cleaner on the glass table right next to Jensen while he was sleeping. On that same day, our house was being cleaned. Although I suggested to the women who did our cleaning that they use nontoxic products, they said that those products were both ineffective and too expensive. (Later in this chapter, I will share some solutions to the problem of toxic household cleansers. Natural products *do* work and they even match the effectiveness of commercial brands. In many cases they are less expensive.)

After these two new exposures, Jensen started wheezing again. Using the Albuterol treatments, we kept his airway clear enough for him to breathe through the night, but by the middle of the night it was clear he needed oxygen. We raced off to the emergency room.

When we were still ten minutes away from the hospital, Jensen stopped breathing and started turning blue. We stopped at the volunteer fire station and started banging on the door. We woke up the firemen who were able to save his life with quick access to oxygen. It was unbelievable to me how quickly Jensen went from okay breathing to no breathing and then to blue—in just minutes! There is no way he would have made it to the hospital.

We spent that night in the hospital, and Jensen was back on antibiotics for pneumonia and doing okay. The next problem was that, although they opened his airways enough to maintain his ability to breathe for short periods of time, they left his airways irritated. The more irritated they were the more reactive mucus he produced. The mucus blocked his bronchioles and caused him to start wheezing. It was then that I realized the medicines that clearly saved his life could take him only so far. In fact, if we overused the Albuterol treatments, we would run the risk of making him worse. So we were stuck in a catch-22, between the life-saving ability of modern medicine and the side effects that perpetuated the problem.

It became painfully clear why there are so many children with asthma who have become dependent on their inhalers. In fact, since 1980, asthma has increased by an alarming 600% in America alone. If we didn't figure something out soon to treat the cause of his condition, Jensen would be sentenced to Albuterol treatments and inhalers for his entire childhood and maybe his life. We tried herbal treatments, which worked for a while but were ultimately too harsh for 9-month-old Jensen.

We struggled for weeks trying to balance herbal treatments and drugs. At first I used the standard herbal asthma formulations, but they did absolutely nothing for him. Most of these herbs have astringent qualities that dry out the mucous membranes. So often in natural medicine we see herbs used in the allopathic tradition, simply as natural alternatives to drugs used to eradicate symptoms. In many cases this can be effective as the herbs work without the side effects of many pharmaceuticals. But, when used allopathically in this way, herbal treatments rarely get to the source of the problem and the cause of the imbalance. The treatments may remove excess mucus while irritating the mucous membranes. These treatments yield symptomatic relief, but just like the Albuterol, they can make the underlying condition even worse.

While we were searching for a more effective and natural treatment to heal and soothe Jensen's irritated respiratory mucous membranes, we started removing allergens in the house with a vengeance. Jensen's first two breathing emergencies came after he had been exposed to cleaning chemicals. This made us suspect that Jensen might be environmentally and chemically sensitive.

At that time, we had a dog at home who was our number-one contributor to indoor air pollution. Jensen was crawling constantly and inhaling the dog's dander and hair into his lungs with every breath. Imagine the size of Jensen's extremely small, 9-month-old bronchioles. Some dog dander, a little dust, and maybe some fur, all of which lie silently on the floor, easily fill up those small spaces. No matter how often and how well the floors and carpets were cleaned, the dog dander was impossible to remove completely. At the time, with Jensen's life on the line, we, as a family, decided to give the dog away. We then cleaned the house, removing of all the possible allergens from top to bottom.

This process involved many steps. We purchased a new vacuum with an excellent filtration system that did not put any of the dust or allergens back into the air. We had our carpets cleaned, and we blew all the house vents out. We hired a company that hooked up a large, powerful vacuum cleaner to all the vents in the house and sucked them clean. It is more common than not that during house construction the workers use the heating vents as garbage holes in which to sweep all the construction dust, debris, and trash. Having the vents vacuumed out was a difficult and expensive process, but it was well worth it. The vent-cleaning company told us that our home had the dirtiest vents they had ever seen.

We continued our quest to make our home allergen-free by purchasing hypo-allergenic mattress and pillow covers for all the beds and pillows in the house (these can be purchased at any bath and bedroom supply store). To be on the safe side, we stopped using feather pillows in Jensen's room, even though the hypo-allergenic pillow covers should have been sufficient to protect him. We bought two electrostatic-type air filters from Sharper Image. These have been phenomenal. Normally, the electrodes in these filters need to be cleaned once every two weeks. But, even with all the cleaning we had been doing, ours needed to be cleaned every two days. Our house was extremely toxic and we didn't know it.

We threw away every toxic chemical and cleaning agent under the sink and in the closets. We replaced all the cleaning products and detergents with natural products. Happily, when we quarantined little Jensen in our new toxin-free home he started improving.

Lesson Two: If your child is struggling with recurring colds or allergies, become an environmental detective. Check your house for allergens and replace all your household cleaners with natural biodegradable and non-toxic cleaners and detergents. These household poisons can be lethal to children like Jensen who have reactive airways. Fortunately, there are many safe products on the market for you to switch to.

Finally, we gave Jensen regular doses of chewable acidophilus and bifidis, two probiotic products that replace the beneficial symbiotic bacteria in the intestines typically killed by antibiotics.

We also gave him multiple doses of powdered and chewable colostrum. Colostrum is the first lactate from a mother's breast milk. It activates a child's immune system. Bovine sources have also been proven to act as powerful immune-boosting agents in humans. Colostrum boosts the immune system and has the typical properties of most dairy products as it is moist, lubricating, and soothing. Most of the allopathic pharmaceutical and herbal treatments prescribed for Jensen by doctors were drying herbs or drugs like Albuterol given to help eliminate excess mucus. They only irritated his already-raw mucous membranes. Shortly after taking each drying agent he got immediately worse. The colostrum provided the perfect combination of immune-building and lubricating properties. It seemed to both lubricate and heal his mucous membranes.

Once the dryness was soothed, his mucous membranes stopped producing excessive reactive mucus and the cause of the problem was finally addressed. Jensen quickly regained his health, and now, almost three years later, he's as healthy as can be. He has had no further episodes of wheezing or breathing difficulty. The couple of colds he has gotten he has beaten in just two or three days on his own. If we did not intervene, today Jensen would be a diagnosed as an asthmatic and allergic child. As many kids are, he would be dependent on inhalers and Albuterol treatments to breathe. It took a team effort—antibiotics, modern medicine, Pat Frazier, non-toxic cleaners, and natural medicines—to bring Jensen back into balance.

Lesson Three: Never underestimate the life-saving power of modern medicine. But there is one caution to keep in mind. Many drugs can aggravate the cause of a condition, making it difficult later to get off the medicine. It may require a joint effort from both allopathic and holistic practitioners to bring your child back to drug-free good health after they've been sick. Build a team of health care providers you trust, now, before your child gets sick.

The Chemical Hit List

Today, children are exposed to chemicals and have levels of toxicity from birth that their parents did not have until they were adults. This means they have more time to develop environmentally triggered diseases with long latency periods such as cancer. In the past 20 to 30 years more and more toxic chemicals have been introduced into the environment. As a result, the level of toxins stored in the fat cells of our bodies has risen. Bio-accumulation studies have shown that some toxins are stored in the body for life. Greater and greater amounts of these are being stored at younger and younger ages.

> A State of Massachusetts study in 1989 reported that 50% of all illness is due to poor indoor air quality.

One study showed that the toxic chemical 1,4-Dichlorobenzene was found in the fat cells of 100% of the people tested. This chemical is found in almost all household deodorizers and room-fresheners and is an example of a seemingly benign product that is rarely touched and never ingested, only inhaled.

Warning labels on containers typically refer to toxic hazards from ingestion. However, only 10% of the health problems related to toxic chemicals are caused by ingestion, while 90% are caused by the inhalation of vapors and absorption of particles. Few people realize that through the inhalation process these chemicals can enter the bloodstream in just a few seconds. Unlike the digestive system, which has an opportunity to break down and dilute the ingested toxin, the airways are the most vulnerable part of the body when exposed to toxic chemicals.

The inhalation of toxic chemicals can be particularly insidious, as some products release contaminants into the air right away while others do so gradually over a period of time. There are many chemicals that can remain in the air for up to a year. According to the American Lung Association, the contaminants found in many household and personal-care products can cause dizziness; nausea; allergic reactions; eye, skin, and respiratory tract irritations; and even cancer.

Bad Guys

The following "Bad-Guy List" includes the most common chemicals to be avoided when buying household and personal-care products. It comes from the book *Clean House, Clean Planet,* by Karen Logan. This book is a "must read" for every parent. It not only explains what to avoid but tells you how to make your own simple, easy, and non-toxic household products at home in less time and with less money than if you purchase them at a store.

The "Bad-Guy List" of ingredients to avoid:

- Alcohol
- Bleach
- Ammonia
- Butyl cellosolve
- Cresol
- Dye
- Ethanol
- Formaldehyde
- Glycols
- Hydrochloric acid
- Hydrofluoric acid
- Lye
- Naphthalene
- NTAs (nitrilotriacetic acid)
- PDCBs (paradichlorobenzenes)
- Perchloroethylene
- Petroleum distillates
- Phenol
- Phosphoric acid
- Phosphates
- Propellants
- Sulfuric acid
- TCE (trichloroethylene)

Imagine a pillowcase, sheets, and pajamas all washed in detergents full of bleach, phosphates, and other respiratory irritants. Your children are breathing these toxins into their lungs, where they enter the bloodstream with each breath. Children breathe, on average, at least 26,000 breaths a day. While asleep, every night, they are breathing in the neighborhood of 10,000 detergent-filled breaths. It is amazing that more children do not react to their significant exposure to these toxins in a violent manner. But more of them may be reacting than we realize. As I mentioned in Chapter 3, children already contract 6 to 8 colds a year and visit the doctor 23 times during the first four years of life. In these visits, respiratory ailments are the most common complaint. We may see more serious reactions show up as our children get older since new studies report that childhood exposure to these chemicals could take years to reveal their health consequences.

How Clean Is Your Laundry?

Even though the NTAs commonly found in laundry detergents are a suspected carcinogen, they are still allowed in laundry soaps. Most commercial laundry detergents leave a caustic film or residue of oily fabric softeners, chemical perfumes, and dyes. Are the clothes that come out of the washing machine really clean?

"Bad-Guy List" phosphates are used in detergents to soften the water and enhance cleaning performance, but are dangerous for both our health and the health of the environment. Phosphates were one of the major contributors to the virtual death of Lake Erie in the 1970s as well as the pollution of many of America's rivers.

Don't be fooled by manufacturers who are now using low-phosphate detergents and marketing themselves as environmentally friendly. In most cases, the phosphates have been replaced with caustic chemicals like lye or potassium hypochlorite. Although these alternatives may be somewhat safer for the environment, they are 100 times more caustic and dangerous to us than phosphates. When swallowed, lye will quickly eat through the esophagus. If accidentally splashed in the eyes, it can cause blindness. It is extremely poisonous yet commonly found in tub and tile, toilet bowl, oven, and drain cleaners, as well as some detergents.

Carcinogens in Your Cabinets

According to the National Cancer Prevention Coalition, the Top 5 cancer-causing products found in the average home are:

- Johnson & Johnson Baby Powder with Talc
- Crest Tartar Control toothpaste
- VO5 Hair Conditioner
- Clairol Nice 'n' Easy hair color
- Ajax cleanser
- Lysol disinfectant

Of the 884 chemicals in personal-care products that were found to be toxic, according to United States House of Representatives reports in 1989:

- 146 cause tumors
- 218 cause reproductive complaints
- 778 cause acute toxicity
- 314 cause biological mutations
- 376 cause skin and eye irritations

Some of these toxic chemicals, such as bleach, which are benignly labeled as disinfectants, are in fact classified as pesticides under the Federal Hazardous Substances Act. According to a State of California study, 40% of the 2,435 pesticide poisonings in one year were due to exposure to disinfectants like the bleach used in household cleaning products. Since the introduction of these pesticides into household cleaning products, childhood cancer rates have increased by 28%. When these cleaners containing bleach are mixed with cleaners containing ammonia, a toxic chloramine gas is produced. This toxic gas can cause coughing, voice loss, feelings of burning or suffocation, and even death.

Some states are taking proactive roles in reducing the amount of toxins found in certain household products. The State of California recently passed legislation requiring a 45% reduction in toxins found in:

- hairspray
- furniture polish
- window cleaners
- air fresheners
- shaving cream
- laundry detergents
- nail polish remover
- insect repellents
- hairstyling gel and mousse

Remove Immediately from Your House

Government regulations require that only the most extremely toxic substances carry a warning label. One of the most common toxic products easily accessible to children, surprisingly, is dishwasher detergent. Its typical location under the sink provides any child with easy access. In one case, a child placed her finger in a full dishwasher soap, and then, as most kids do, she put her finger in her mouth. The small amount of soap on her finger burned holes through her esophagus. It took five operations to repair the damage from one finger-full of liquid dishwasher soap. There is an "extreme warning" label on the back of dishwasher soap, but very few people take the time to read it. When it comes to your child's health, put safety first and remove from your home any product containing one of the "extreme warning" labels required by the government.

Remove products with these labels from your home:

- "Do not induce vomiting"
- "Corrosive—irritates skin immediately"
- "Call physician immediately"
- "Harmful or fatal if swallowed"

- "Warning!" (As little as one teaspoon can harm or kill an adult.)
- "Danger!" (As few as five drops can harm or kill an adult.)

When To Get Help

Know your local poison control center number and have it posted by the phone—or programmed into one of the speed-dial options. Play it safe and call the American Association of Poison Control Centers (800.222.1222) whenever your child has swallowed something that should not have been ingested.

According to an article in the November 2001 issue of *Ladies' Home Journal*, if you find your child near an open cabinet full of cleaning supplies but you're not sure what—if anything—was swallowed, smell the child's mouth, face, and clothes. If you detect anything suspicious or are simply unsure, call poison control. **Get immediate help if you notice any of the signs of poisoning, which include: staggering walk, vomiting, and excessive sleeping.** *Never* induce vomiting without the advice of poison control. Substances like bleach and drain cleaners which burn the esophagus on the way down can also cause burns on the way back up.

 Parental Tip: Know your poison control center number and have it posted by your phone, programmed into speed dial...and programmed into your cell phone.

Formaldehyde—A Silent Killer

Formaldehyde is a highly toxic chemical and known cancer-causing agent. It damages the neurological tissue in the body and irritates the eyes, nose, throat, and lungs. Because it irritates the mucous membranes in the respiratory system, it often triggers the chronic production of excessive mucus. This excessive mucus disarms the immune system in its ability to prevent and fight infections. One in five people are known to be hypersensitive to formaldehyde.

Formaldehyde is commonly found in:

- pharmaceutical drugs
- mouthwash
- hairspray
- cosmetics
- cleaning products
- perfumes
- waxes
- hairstyling lotions
- shampoo
- air fresheners
- fungicides
- fingernail polish
- floor polishes
- dry-cleaning solvents
- toothpaste
- laundry spray starch
- antiperspirants
- glues and adhesives
- particle board
- carpet glues
- ...and many more

American children are constantly exposed to formaldehyde. One source of exposure is off-gassing from the particleboard that has replaced plywood to build homes and construct furniture. It is rare today to find a home that is free of furniture made with particleboard, whose most common adhesive is urea-formaldehyde.

One of the many health conditions linked to formaldehyde is ADHD, or attention deficit hyperactivity disorder, the incidence of which has risen significantly in American children over the last ten years. Associated with this rise is the increased use of formaldehyde in household, personal-care, and building products. In 1993, for example, 4.5 million children in the U.S. used the drug Ritalin in order to be able to sit still long enough to learn. By 1998, 11.4 million children in the U.S. were taking this powerful Class 2 narcotic drug, according the *Detroit News* in March of 1998. (Class 2 narcotics are restricted substances that can be habit-forming and illegal to possess without a written prescription.) ADHD is not the only condition linked to the use of formaldehydes.

Some of the others are:

- skin reactions
- ear infections
- headaches
- depression
- asthma
- joint pain
- dizziness
- mental confusion
- nausea
- disorientation
- phlebitis
- fatigue
- vomiting
- sleep disturbances
- laryngitis
- cancers, especially in the nasal passages where formaldehyde vapors are inhaled

Formaldehyde Hidden in Labels

To be sure that you're not using formaldehyde products in your home, here is a list of alternate names commonly used for the formaldehyde family of chemicals. If you see any of these names in products, know that you are exposing your family to the toxic effects of formaldehyde.

Avoid using products with any of these ingredients:

- Bfv
- Fannoform

- Formalin
- Formalin 40
- Formalith
- Formic Aldehyde
- Formol
- Fyde
- Hoch
- Ivalon
- Karsan
- Lysoform
- Methaldehyde
- Methanal
- Methyl Aldehyde
- Methylene Glycol
- Methylene Oxide
- Morbocid
- Oxomethane
- Oxymethlene
- Paraform
- Polyoxmethylene
- Trioxane

Phenol—Another Silent Toxin

Carbolic acid is a type of phenol (a very large group of chemicals, some dangerous, others are beneficial) which is extremely caustic and burns the skin with external exposure. If ingested or inhaled it can cause: damage to the central nervous system, pneumonia, respiratory tract infections, heart rate irregularities, skin irritations, kidney and liver damage, numbness, vomiting, and even death. Fortunately, many manufacturers have recently started substituting for carbolic acid with less toxic derivatives.

Carbolic acid is commonly found in products including:

- air fresheners
- aftershave

- bronchial mists
- Chloroseptic throat spray
- deodorants
- hairspray
- decongestants
- mouthwash
- aspirin
- acne medications
- antiseptics
- calamine lotions
- detergents
- hairstyling lotions
- cold capsules
- all-purpose cleaners
- anti-itch lotions
- sunscreens
- cough syrup
- cosmetics
- hand lotions
- …and many more

Read the labels of all personal care and cleaning products to be sure!!!

Internet Resources to Learn more about Chemicals in the Home

- *www.epa.gov/opptintr/kids/hometour.htm*
- *www.bygpub.com/natural/living.htm*
- *www.consumerlawpage.com/article/household-chemicals.shtml*
- *www.oprah.com/tows/pastshows/tows_2002tows_past_20020531_c.jhtml*
- *www.usatoday.com/news/health/spotlight/2001-11-08-chec.htm*
- *www.checnet.org*
- *Or contact me at www.LifeSpa.com*

Environment and Health-Conscious Product Companies

The following companies offer environmentally safe and health-conscious cleaning products through catalogs or direct sales. Co-ops in your area are also a great source for these often expensive products.

Seventh Generation
49 Hercules Drive
Colchester, VT 05446
800.456.1177
www.seventhgeneration.com

Real Goods
555 Leslie Street
Ukiah, CA 95482
800.762.7325
www.realgoods.com

Washington Toxics Coalition
4516 University Way NE
Seattle, WA 98105
206.632.1545

Bio-Integral Resource Center
P.O. Box 7414
Berkeley, CA 94707
510.524.2567
(for pest control)

Melaleuca
Idaho Falls, ID 83401
800.282.3000
www.melaleuca.com

SafeScience
31 St. James Avenue
Boston, MA 02116
866.SAFE.SCI

The cheapest and safest way to remove toxic chemicals and ingredients from your home is to make your own cleaning products. Many cleaning products can be made safely with simple, non-toxic ingredients that work extremely effectively.

Some of the best resources I have found include:

- Karen Logan, *Clean House, Clean Planet* (Pocket Books, 1997).
- Shirley Camper Soman, *Let's Stop Destroying Our Children* (Hawthorne Books, 1974).
- Debra Lynn Dadd, *The Non-Toxic Home and Office* (Jeremy Tarcher, 1992).
- Joyce Shoemaker, Ph.D. & Charity Vitale, Ph.D., *Healthy Homes, Healthy Kids* (Island Press, 1991).

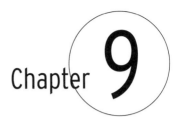

Chapter 9

Secret 8—Inspection!!!

As you realize by now, the seeds of susceptibility to a cold or other illness are sown days, weeks, and even months before it arrives. These signs of vulnerability are publicly announced by your child's body; you just need to be aware of their presence. In this chapter, I map out a list of the most important "cold prevention tips" so you can employ therapeutic measures to stop a cold it in its tracks at the very first sign of its arrival. I will also describe how the onset of a cold can be caused by the seeds of imbalance sown a season or two prior.

Understanding who your children are and during which season they are particularly vulnerable gives you valuable tools to help prevent colds and reduce susceptibilities to getting sick, thereby maintain optimal health for your children.

> **In Ayurvedic medicine, cold prevention is a way of life.** Understanding a child's constitution, or kid-type, and how he or she is impacted by the seasons is important information for parents to use in order to adjust diet, sleeping patterns, lifestyle, exercise, and herbs to ensure that their child does not get sick.

Before the discovery of penicillin in 1929 and the wide use of antibiotic drugs beginning in the 1940s, many conditions like pneumonia, deep lung congestion, pertussis, and diphtheria were life-threatening, especially for children. Today, we have antibiotics to bail us out when children become ill with an infection. Before these drugs were available, even though many herbs also have antibiotic effects, *prevention* of serious illnesses was the most effective form of treatment. Traditional medical systems, including Ayurveda, were based on the rules of prevention and emphasized treating individuals while they were still healthy in order to maintain their health rather than waiting until they became sick.

Different Susceptibilities

Ayurvedic medicine describes how different kid-types have varying levels of vulnerability to getting sick in different seasons of the year or times in their lives. Being aware of these can make the difference between your child coming down with cold after cold in the winter or dripping with a runny nose all spring. I will describe the Ayurvedic tools used to identify high-risk activities or times of the year, how to treat the initial signs of a cold days or weeks before it actually arrives, and how to treat children when they are healthy.

Secret Eight: The eighth secret is knowing how to treat your children when they are healthy and when they are at greater risk to getting sick. Knowing your children's constitutions and watching for changes in their behavior, appearance, elimination, sleep, and other habits can reveal underlying imbalances before they manifest as illness. By inspecting your children regularly, knowing what to look for, and then adjusting their diet, supplements, or other activities, you can make cold- and illness-prevention a way of life.

Summer Kid-Type Risk

Knowing that your child is a hot summer kid-type who is vulnerable to becoming overheated in the summer months is critical for preventing bouts of illness during the cold and flu season. Throughout

the summer months, nature provides a buffet of cooling foods
that appease summer kid-types.
If the heat of summer kid-types
is not kept at bay in the summer
months, the excess accumulated

> Keeping the Summer kid-type cool in the summer is the key to preventing illness in the fall, winter and spring.

heat will dry them out, making their mucous membranes especially
vulnerable to and irritated by the severe dryness of the winter season.
The result, of course, is excess mucus production in children who,
during this time of their lives, make mucus for a living. This then
leads to the cascading effect I have discussed throughout the book.

To prevent summer kid-types from succumbing to illness in the
winter cold and flu season and to allergies and asthma in the spring,
parents must employ preventive techniques months in advance—in
the heat of the summer.

Summer Kid-Type Preventive Techniques

1. Strictly choose foods from the summer grocery list in the
   summer months (details in Chapter 7).
2. At the end of summer when the heat is more intense,
   increase the portions of cooling fruits like apples, melons,
   pomegranates, and bitter greens.
3. As summer ends, follow the winter diet carefully in the fall
   and winter months to counter the tendency toward becoming
   dried out.
4. Getting proper rest is crucial, especially during the long
   nights of winter, for the high-energy constitution of a
   summer kid-type.
5. Their natural tendency to become overheated makes them
   the most likely candidates to become dehydrated. To keep
   hydrated, they (any kid-type, but especially summer kid-
   types) must drink 1/2 their body weight in ounces of pure
   water daily. This is above and beyond any soda pop, juice, or
   other liquids (details in Chapter 5).
6. Follow the cold-prevention tips outlined in this chapter. For

example, take chywanprash, an herbal jam described later on in this chapter on page 245, during the summer months and toward summer's end to increase immunity, and reduce excessive heat and dryness.

Winter Kid-Type Risk

The winter kid-type has a different set of vulnerabilities from the summer kid-type. While winter kid-types do not run as great a risk of becoming overheated in the summer, they do have a increased susceptibility to becoming dried out. We have all noticed the tendency for the sinuses and skin to dry out toward the end of the summer. But winter kid-types tend to dry out faster than anyone else, leading to excess mucus production, causing them to run an even higher risk of coming down with a cold or flu in the winter months.

> The key to cold prevention in Winter kid-types is to keep them from becoming excessively dried out.

The soothing, comforting, and lubricating winter harvest is the winter kid-type's most important medicine. Of all the seasonal diets, winter kid-types should follow the winter diet the most strictly. If your child seems to be excessively dry in late summer, start choosing foods from the winter grocery list in September or October rather than waiting until November. Starting the winter diet a little early will help to get a head start on keeping the skin and mucous membranes moist and lubricated during cold and flu season.

Winter Kid-Type Preventive Techniques

1. Start eating foods from the winter grocery list early, in September or October (details in Chapter 7).
2. Follow the winter grocery lists strictly throughout the winter months.
3. Keep your house humid with cool mist humidifiers in the winter. Steam humidifiers breed and disseminate bacteria, while cool mists are less likely to do so.

4. Keep the skin from getting dried out using the oil massage described in Chapter 3.

5. Carefully follow the cold-prevention tips in this chapter. For example, give fall- and winter-harvested ashwaganda prophylactically in the winter—especially toward the end of the season when the cold and dryness are more intense (see Chapter 10).

Spring Kid-Type Risk

Unlike the summer and winter kid-types, spring kid-types rarely dry out. They are the thoroughbreds of mucus makers. Summer comes just in time for spring kid-types to help heat up and dry out the excessive mucus that accumulates in their bodies in the spring.

The typically dry winter months do not have the same drying effect on the skin and mucous membranes of a spring kid-type as they do on a summer or winter kid-type. Spring kid-types have a natural immunity to becoming dry and do not need an excuse to make mucus at any time of year—it is their nature. These spring kid-types are more susceptible to coughs, asthma, allergies, and chronic colds, primarily due to their natural tendency to make more mucus. While spring kid-types will not be at *severe* risk until the rains, moisture, and muddiness of spring set in, they are always at risk due to their production of excessive cold-causing mucus.

To prevent colds, parents have to be careful not to feed their spring kid-type children highly mucus-producing foods at any time of year. But the wet spring season is when parents need to be the most vigilant.

Because children are in their spring lifecycle, it will clearly be spring kid-types who will be the most challenging to keep healthy. When spring kid-types reach their teens and enter the summer lifecycle they will begin to flourish. The summer lifecycle, like the summer season, provides relief for the spring

> The dryness, warmth, and sun of summer are typically therapeutic for the wet, heavy, mucusy Spring kid-types.

kid-type. Nature is on the side of spring kid-types in their summer lifecycle; in this time of their life their tendency to make mucus and their susceptibility to colds, allergies, and asthma will dramatically decrease. There is light at the end of the tunnel for the spring kid-type!

This does not mean that it is impossible to keep your spring kid-type child healthy. On the contrary, once you realize the susceptibilities of the spring kid-type you can employ preventive techniques on a regular basis. Here is a list of preventive suggestions for the spring kid-type:

Spring Kid-Type Preventive Techniques

1. Reduce mucus-producing foods in the winter and spring.
2. Eating moderate amounts of mucus-producing foods in the hot summer is okay.
3. Rarely or never eat mucus-producing foods at nighttime.
4. Eat supper as early as possible (details in Chapter 6).
5. If by chance, they eat a late supper, supplement their digestive system with trikatu, which reduces mucus production (details in Chapters 4 and 7).
6. Closely follow the spring grocery list in the spring and focus on eating greens and drinking green drinks daily (details in Chapter 7).
7. Encourage your spring kid-type child to get more exercise and avoid being sedentary (details in Chapter 11).
8. Start the spring diet as early as late February (depending on the climate in your area).
9. With spring kid-types, early detection of a cold is the best medicine. Follow the cold-prevention tips in this chapter carefully. For example, take turmeric, which is spring-harvested, in this time of year to keep excessive mucus production at bay.

Daily Inspection

It is important for parents to actively look for and be able to recognize the warning signs of a brewing cold days before it actually arrives. When something is not quite right, our bodies continually send messages in the form of early signs and symptoms. It is crucial to learn how to observe the body and to recognize what is significant. This can be tricky; although most signs are very obvious, others are more subtle. Early detection is the best cold prevention.

Early Morning

Children might wake up sneezing, with puffy eyes or a slight cough or runny nose. If you ask them how they feel, they will almost always say "fine." But

> Many of the key signs of a cold looming on the horizon are seen in the first morning hours after rising.

these are the very first signs of an infection that you must recognize and treat early to avoid a full-blown cold or a case of the flu.

Some important questions to ask yourself are: Are my children exhausted when they get up? Do they have circles under their eyes? If it is early winter, check them for excessive dry skin as this can be a precursor to a weakened immune system. Check their elimination and their appetite. Is the problem originating in the respiratory system, upper-digestive system, or in their eliminative system? Once you finish the inspection, you can make on-the-spot dietary adjustments, a technique I teach in the next chapter using the Lazy Susan of cold prevention.

The Runny Nose

Even though it seems contradictory to think of a wet, mucusy runny rose as being "dry," a runny nose is usually caused by dryness and irritation in the sinuses. In the early stages of a runny nose, you can usually get away with giving the child drying herbs to arrest the symptoms. Most over-the-counter cold remedies work in this way, through drying out the sinuses. But if the mucous membranes are already dry and irritated then treatments aimed at lubricating and soothing the mucous membranes will yield the most effective and permanent results. The Ayurvedic approach offers herbal therapies that restore balance by simultaneously liquefying the mucus and healing the irritated mucous membranes.

Before I describe treatments for a runny nose, let's talk about the signs children will exhibit even before the nose starts to run. Usually, days before the runny nose starts, you'll hear a nasal tone in their voice first thing in the morning. Additionally, their face often becomes puffy, and the area under their eyes becomes swollen and slightly darker. This imbalance could be due to a seasonal change, being run-down, too much pizza and Mac 'n' Cheese late at night, recently returning from a trip, or an excess of stress in their life.

At this onset stage of a runny nose there are a variety of effective treatments. And fortunately, this early in the game, a cold is much less tenacious and easy to treat. Let's review two treatments for runny noses that we mentioned in previous chapters:

Turmeric—to help liquefy mucus and soothe the beginnings of a sinus or mucous membrane inflammation. Mix equal parts of turmeric and raw honey into a paste, and take 1 teaspoon of the paste one to three times a day, depending on how early in the cold's lifecycle you are treating it. In some cases, as little as one dose of the turmeric paste can reverse a runny nose. Tumeric is a great preventive treatment for the spring cold and allergy season; it is harvested in the spring as an aid to liquefying and removing excess cold-causing mucus.

Trikatu—a combination of black pepper, long pepper, and ginger. Mix equal parts of trikatu with raw honey into a paste. Use more honey if necessary to make it taste palatable to a child. Take 1/2 teaspoon of the paste one to three times a day or as needed to reverse the cold. Trikatu is specific for upper-respiratory conditions.

A Spoonful of Sugar
Another herb to use before a cold begins, or even after it has become

full-blown is chywanprash. Chywanprash is one of my long-time favorite cold-preventers. I have used it with great success for years with my own kids and with my patients—children and adults.

Aaron was an 8-year-old boy whose mom brought him to see me because he was experiencing a series of chronic colds, one right after another. The countless cycles of antibiotics Aaron took only made him worse, and his chronic colds continued. Aaron was frustrated and tired of being sick. He was run-down, exhausted, thin, and had dark circles under his eyes. It was clear that Aaron needed both support to fight his colds and restore balance to his irritated mucous membranes and physical strengthening and rejuvenation to help his body recover from exhaustion and resist infection.

When Aaron came to see me, his mom told me that he was in the beginning stages of yet another cold. They were hoping I could do something to turn this cold around. I gave Aaron a jar of chywanprash—an herbal jam—and I offered to make him a deal: I told him that if he could finish this jar in one week I would give him five dollars. His eyes popped out of his head. "Not only will I give you five dollars if you finish the jar," I told him, "but you will not catch the cold that is knocking on your door." His mother smiled in approval of my unorthodox plan.

I told him that this stuff didn't taste great, but that it wasn't terrible either. It has a consistency like peanut butter and a sweet, sour, and tart taste.

We shook hands and off he went. About two weeks later, my secretary knocked on my door while I was with a patient and told me, "There is a little kid out here that says you made a bet with him and you owe him five dollars." I walked outside to see Aaron with a smile on his face that stretched from ear to ear.

"So you finished the jar of goop?" (Goop is what the kids call it.)

"Yup!" he answered.

"Did you get a cold?"

"Nope!"

"So I guess I owe you five dollars?"

"Yup."

He was so proud of himself. I gave him the five dollars, his mother bought another jar of chywanprash, and off they went well on their way to breaking the cycle of recurring colds.

Chywanprash is an amazing natural multi-mineral and multi-vitamin formulation (though it doesn't the have recommended daily dosages of every vitamin and mineral) with powerful free radical scavenging properties. It contains more than 40 herbs, with one herb providing the base and main ingredient. That base herb is the citrus fruit called *amalaki*, Indian Gooseberry (*Emblica officinalis*). It is also one of the three fruits in trifala (described in Chapter 4). Each fruit contains more than 3 grams of completely bio-available Vitamin C; this is a greater level of Vitamin C pound-for-pound than any other plant yet discovered. Amalaki is harvested in the summer, giving it cooling properties. It is also one of the most powerful rejuvenative herbs used in Ayurveda.

The story of the development of chywanprash comes from one of the original Vedic textbooks, dating from over 3,000 years ago. It was originally developed to restore health and youthfulness to an elderly man named Chyawan—from which the herbal formula got its name. When Chyawan was in his 90s, he met a very young woman whom he fell in love with. He was desperate to find a way to restore his youth so he could enjoy a full life with his newfound love. In his quest, Chyawan went to the most revered Ayurvedic doctors of the time and requested an herbal formulation to restore his youth.

They came up with a formula they labeled chywanprash, "eaten by Chyawan." The story goes that Chyawan did restore his youth, married his young bride, and even started a family.

The original formula has been passed down and kept alive for over 3,000 years (significantly longer than any modern pharmaceutical medication in use today). It is one of the most popular and widely used formulations in Ayurvedic medicine.

This formula has many powerful effects. It is rejuvenating—for Aaron it helped him build up his strength, stamina and immunity. Thanks to its high natural Vitamin C content, it is an effective cold-fighter. It also contains a variety of peppers hidden within the formula that have actions similar to that of trikatu's ability to liquefy mucus and fight upper sinus infections. Because it is

> Kids in India today take a teaspoon of chywanprash each morning they way American kids take Flintstones vitamins.

prepared as an herbal jam and cooked for two to three days prior to use, it is predigested and well broken down, making it easy to assimilate by people of all ages, including children or the elderly.

My own kids take chywanprash on a regular basis—usually only 1 teaspoon in the morning, about three times a week, when they're healthy. If they are showing signs of fatigue, stress, or a brewing cold, I'll give them a lot more. Chywanprash can be taken safely in large doses, even by children; it's more a food than a medicine.

> My 12-year-old came home recently complaining of a scratchy throat and feeling achy and tired. I gave her a jar of chywanprash, a spoon, a large glass of water, and instructions to drink the water and eat 6 teaspoons of goop. The next morning she woke up ready to go with no cold in sight.

The cooling summer-harvested citrus fruit amalaki is a perfect antidote during the summer and at summer's end for the cold-causing risk factors of accumulated heat and dryness.

Parental Tip: Using chywanprash at the end of the hot summer season can help prevent end-of-summer colds and allergies, making the back-to-school days much safer and healthier for your child. In fall and winter, the herbal goop will help protect everyone in the house from the dreaded cold and flu season. Eating chywanprash in the spring helps to liquefy and clear out built up mucus and strengthens the body during the wet, damp season. Chywanprash can be eaten throughout the year for constant cold protection and boosting of the immune system.

Those Unsightly Dark Circles

Some children have a tendency to get dark circles under their eyes. These are important physical symptoms to notice, as they can give information about conditions beneath the surface. Some kids get them only when they are run-down, tired, and exhausted, while others seem to have them all the time. Dark circles are a sign of poor circulation, especially the lymphatic drainage of the head and neck. Due to dryness and poor circulation, the waste is unable to move out of the head and will accumulate and then be stored in the tissues beneath the eyes.

These dark circles are almost always due to an inability to remove waste properly. Dark circles that appear only at the onset of a cold can be remedied with herbs to lubricate the sinuses, flush the lymphatic system, and increase circulation.

It is said that the eyes are the windows to the soul, but the condition of the area around the eyes can be indicative of the general health of the waste removal system in the body. When your children have chronic dark circles under their eyes, the kidneys could be a factor. In this case, one of the first questions to ask is: "How is my child's hydration?" (See Chapter 5.) Elimination is also a concern with the appearance of chronic dark circles. Because of the direct relationship between the large intestine and the liver via the enteric cycle (the blood from the large intestine drains into the portal system which takes the impurities directly to the liver), many conditions of the liver are treated effectively by restoring proper function to the large intestine and improving elimination. Be a detective. Has there been a chronic constipation problem, history of stomachaches, sore throats, or rashes? These signs may point you in the direction of eliminative concerns.

These conditions, if left alone, can create bigger problems down the road. As parents, we can always be involved in restoring health to our children. By treating some of these chronic conditions you may be addressing underlying concerns that could predispose your child to a more severe liver or kidney condition later in life. Again, prevention is a child's best medicine.

Whenever your child has a chronic condition, you must get an appropriate diagnosis and rule out any serious concerns. Treating liver and kidney issues is outside the scope of this book and is best dealt with by your primary health care provider.

Echinacea

Echinacea is one of the best herbs for both enhancing the body's immune response and flushing the lymphatic system. To date there has never been a report of an overdose or side effects from the use of echinacea. Echinacea is a well-known cold-fighter, but contrary to what most people think, it is not a strong antibacterial or antiviral agent. In one study echinacea showed antibacterial activity only if 30 drops of the extract were taken every two hours for seven days. This is more often than most people would take it, so they would never get enough to elicit its antibacterial properties.

Echinacea functions primarily by increasing the body's natural ability to fight off a cold, flu, or other illness. Echinacea generally works on the interconnected lymphatic and immune systems; it both increases lymphatic circulation and stimulates the body's production of macrophages, one of the types of white blood cells crucial to healthy functioning of the immune system.

Lymphatic circulation is connected to both hydration (discussed in Chapter 5) and exercise (addressed in Chapter 11). Both of these are crucial to the health and well-being of your child. Lack of proper exercise impedes the flow of fluid in the lymphatic system, so a sedentary child will have a greater risk of developing lymphatic congestion and the resulting colds.

How To Take Echinacea:

Extracts of echinacea are much more effective than capsules or dried herb. More of the active ingredients in echinacea are retained in extracts of fresh herb than in the dried herb. Fortunately, many sweet-tasting fruit- or berry-flavored non-alcoholic glycerin extracts are now available. This is a great resource for parents because children typically like the taste of glycerin extracts better than the taste of alcoholic tinctures.

Echinacea is best taken as early as possible when you suspect a child is coming down with a cold. It can be given often, one eye-dropper-full dose every hour for the first day or two of a cold to enhance lymphatic circulation. If needed, it can be taken for up to seven days for a cold. Once the cold arrives, there are more effective herbs than echinacea to treat it. There is, however, research that supports the cumulative effect of taking echinacea over several days in fighting a cold; so if your child loves the sweet-tasting echinacea extract for kids, as my 3-year-old does, then don't fight it. Use it to resolve your child's condition. As most parents know, if you find something that works and tastes good—it seems too good to be true.

Ear Oil

Lubricating the eustachian tubes is one of the best remedies for dry sinuses and dry or congested cervical lymphatic drainage. The eustachian tubes run parallel to the cervical lymphatic system, so if they dry out, the ears lose their lymphatic drainage. Dry eustachian tubes and subsequent lymphatic stagnation is a common cause of a sore throat.

> One of the best-kept secrets for a healthy child is the use of ear oil.

This combination of symptoms—dry eustachian tubes, compromised lymphatic drainage, and sore throat—leads to irritated mucous membranes and the production of excessive mucus. We now have the perfect breeding ground for an infection in the ears. Ear oils, called *karuna purana* in Ayurveda, can be used as both a preventive technique and as a treatment for earaches, sinus infections, sore throats, and colds.

In our house in the winter, when the dry air brings with it a greater risk of sinuses and cervical lymph becoming dry, I apply ear oil to my children's ears prophylactically once a month, or even as often as once every two weeks if I suspect a cold-in-the-making.

Most ear oils are rich in demulcent herbs like mullein or slippery elm and some have garlic or tea tree oil to help fight an infection. Almost any ear oil will be effective, as the naturally lubricating quality of oil is the key to its success. There are numerous ear oils available at your local health food store, or you can make your own, which is my preference. Typically, I use the following formulation.

How To Make Your Own Ear Oil

1. Start with a clean, empty, dry 1-ounce dropper bottle.
2. Fill the bottle with half castor oil and half olive or cold-pressed sesame oil.
3. Add 10 to 15 drops of garlic oil and shake well.
4. Add 10 to 15 drops of tea tree oil and shake well.

How To Use Ear Oil

1. Shake the bottle of oil well and set it in a cup of hot water in the sink, or run hot water over it to gently warm the oil.
2. Test the oil before using in the ear to make sure it is warm and not hot.
3. While the child is lying on his or her side, or while asleep, fill the ear (filling the canal) with the warm oil.
4. Let the oil sit in the ear for 5 to10 minutes as you massage behind the ear and upper neck with your fingers.
5. Place a cotton ball in the ear and flip the child over, and then repeat the same procedure for the child's other ear.

For several children, you can oil their ears one after the other:

1. Have them each lie on their side while the oil is being heated in the sink.
2. Once the oil is ready you can squirt the oil in each child's ear, filling the canal before the oil cools off.
3. Massage each child's neck and then place a cotton ball in the ear.
4. Flip them all over and repeat the process.

When To Use Ear Oil

- Once to twice a month in the winter to effectively prevent illnesses resulting from dry sinuses and cervical lymph.
- Every night when a child has a cold or earache, until the symptoms are resolved.

Check Your Child's Elimination

 Parental Tip: If your children have dark circles under their eyes that are long-standing and not associated only with the onset of the cold or fatigue, then you need to look at the efficiency of their digestion and elimination.

Knowing the elimination habits of your children is an important part of the inspection process. I can't tell you how often, when I ask about elimination with children and their parents in my office, no one knows the answer. I cannot remember meeting any children who knew off the top of their head how many times a day they moved their bowels. Parents often have a rough idea of their child's eliminative habits but rarely notice if a child skips the daily bowel movement for a day or two. When a child is in the beginning stages of coming down with a cold, changes in elimination patterns are often the first sign that something may be amiss, and parents need to tune into this right away. The best way for parents to keep track of their child's elimination is to get their child on a regular cycle.

Different kid-types will have different normal patterns of elimination. When they are in balance, summer kid-types typically have multiple bowel movements, spring kid-types may have two full and complete eliminations, and the dryer winter kid-types will, we hope, have one full and complete elimination first thing in the morning. I would not expect a winter kid-type to have more than one elimination per day.

> It is extremely difficult to keep track of a child's elimination if it is irregular.

The healthiest pattern for a child or an adult is to move the bowels first thing in the morning. The best and most effective way to ensure morning elimination is to start each day with a large glass of water and a little exercise, yoga, or stretching.

This routine of morning elimination is often dependent on the previous night's dinner. If dinner happened to be pizza at eight o'clock at night, it will be difficult for any kid-type to have a first-thing-in-the-morning elimination. In general, late-night dinners considerably slow the digestive and eliminative cycles. In Chapter 4, I discussed a variety of herbs that can be used to enhance and support the digestive process when eating hard-to-digest late-evening meals. By taking herbs to support the digestive process it is possible for a child to wake up in the morning, and after a large class of water, have a full and complete elimination.

Sometimes it can take weeks for a child with irregular elimination to get back on a first-thing-in-the-morning elimination digestive cycle, but making sure that your child stays on a this cycle is paramount. When the elimination slows down, impurities accumulate in the large intestine and become absorbed into the lymphatic system, ultimately moving into the liver. Once the lymphatic system is overwhelmed, the immune system becomes compromised.

Dark circles under the eyes are connected to dysfunction in the immune, lymphatic, and eliminative systems—and to a greater risk of susceptibility to colds. All of the systems in the body work together in an interconnected fashion. It is for this same reason that exercise and proper hydration are so effective in keeping dark circles away. Understanding how a late dinner can throw this cycle off and how taking some digestive herbs can mitigate late-nights dinner can be incredibly useful in helping your child stay healthy.

> Daily, full, and complete elimination keeps the lymphatic system and the immune system functional and healthy, allowing the body to effectively fight colds and illnesses on its own.

Is Your Child Tired Out and Overworked?

Today, children are often burdened with intense schoolwork and a plethora of after-school activities like sports, theater, music lessons, and play dates, all of which make them susceptible to becoming exhausted. When the body is tired, it treats life as an emergency and shifts into a crisis response. Once the crisis alarm is raised, the body produces excessive amounts of stress-fighting hormones. These hormones increase blood sugar, raise the heart rate, store fat under the mattress, and suppress digestion and the immune system in order to focus the body's energy on fighting the immediate stress. This cascade of effects makes these hormones degenerative by nature. They are also degenerative because they produce free radicals as waste products. free radicals are now suspected to be the leading cause of aging, disease, cancer, and even death.

Many experts now agree that 80% of all disease is caused by stress. The chemistry of stress causes degeneration of the body, depletion of the nervous system, problems with digestion and elimination, and an increased susceptibility to colds, allergies, acute illness, and chronic disease.

Children show their fatigue and stress level in a variety of ways:

- Irritability
- Low tolerance of siblings or other family members
- Talking back
- Difficulty waking up in the morning
- Difficulty settling down to sleep in the evening

Sleepless Nights

Even though children do not typically show the classic signs of insomnia that one may see in an adult, they can exhibit the early signs of sleep disorders. When someone has a difficult time going to sleep or experiences insomnia, the most common solution is to give them a sedative. However, most sleep disorders are not caused by too much energy and being unable to settle down—the symptoms sedatives are designed to address. It is more likely that people with sleep disorders are exhausted and do not have enough energy to settle down. The body draws on its store of reserve energy to produce natural sedative hormones and neurotransmitter levels which relax the body in preparation for sleep. If the body is exhausted, then there is not enough energy to produce these sleep hormones and the body will stay wired and tired.

Over-the-counter sleep aids are sedatives that force the body to sleep, but do not bring true rest. They do not rebalance the natural sedative hormones to create a state of relaxation in the body. Many of the common over-the-counter sedatives are antihistamines, the same chemicals used in cold medications to dry out the mucous membranes. They have the side effect of sedating the nervous system, which is why cold medicines make us tired.

Children so often will experience a desire to stay up later, watch TV, read, and do anything besides going to sleep. Parents need to be aware of this behavior and enforce early bedtimes—even with young teenagers. For high school-age children, the proper bedtime to get a sufficient amount of rest is typically nine or ten o'clock. If your teenager sleeps in on Saturday morning until ten in the morning, that's a sign that he or she is exhausted and not getting adequate rest in the earlier part of the week. The only time the body can really catch up on quality needed sleep is before ten at night.

For most younger kids, getting them to bed by eight o'clock is a goal every parent should aim to reach. Even though you may not be able to get your children to bed by eight o'clock every night, remember the 51% rule. Have them go to bed early more often than late. A good compromise for parents and children is to alternate late nights when schoolwork is intense with early nights when the responsibilities are less. Letting your child stay up late every night will eventually lead to exhaustion that will compromise your child's health.

> When you artificially sedate someone who is already tired and naturally sedated from exhaustion, you may initially make the symptom better, but at the cost of making the cause—the deep state of exhaustion—even worse.

Herbs for Stress

When kids are working hard, in many cases staying up late to finish their homework, it is useful to know some herbs that can provide adaptogenic support. True adaptogens help the body adapt to stress by supporting the immune system, increasing endurance and stabilizing blood sugar levels. Unfortunately, many herbs and compounds on the market labeled as adaptogens are really stimulants in disguise. These stimulants will help the individual feel better, have more energy, and handle more stress, but will do so only temporarily. They fire up an energy supply the body cannot really spare.

It is important for parents to avoid such stimulants as they will only drive their child deeper into exhaustion. I would stay away from anything that is marketed or sold as an energy drink or formula. Another important substance to avoid is caffeinated drinks. Caffeinated sodas are so abundant today, and kids love them. Older kids succumb to the temptation of caffeine as coffee, which is fashionable among the high school crowd. But it is important to do your best to limit these high-sugar content caffeinated drinks.

> When a person takes stimulants it is analogous to going to the bank and borrowing five dollars to make it through the day. If you do this too often, soon you will receive a message from the bank: "We cannot lend you any more money. Your reserves are exhausted, and now it is time to start paying the money back."

There are a few true adaptogens that are effective for helping children stay strong during times of stress. Chywanprash, which I mentioned earlier in this chapter, is one very effective formulation that can help restore and maintain energy without over-stimulating the body. Another adaptogen, another of my favorites, is an herb called *ashwaganda*.

Ashwaganda

The herb ashwaganda, translated as "the strength of ten horses," is commonly called Winter Cherry (*Withania somerifera*). The root of this plant is an amazing adaptogenic herb that can be given to children in the morning to give them enough energy to run a marathon and given again in the evening before bed so they can sleep like a baby. I have not run across any other herb that can both boost energy and relax a person to sleep. This herb is neither a stimulant nor a sedative. It deeply rejuvenates the nervous system, especially the ability to handle stress. At the same time, ashwaganda strengthens the musculoskeletal system to handle the rigors of physical activity. It's so safe that it is typically given during pregnancy to help support a strong and vital mother and baby.

This root herb is part of the fall harvest taken throughout the fall and winter to help rebuild the nervous, immune, and musculoskeletal systems. It can be taken for stress at any time of year with only one caveat—it has a heating effect on the body due to it being a fall- and winter-harvested herb. This makes it good in the fall, winter and spring. It can be used with caution in the summer, and with additional caution with a summer kid-type.

How To Take Ashwaganda
Ashwaganda can be taken first thing in the morning before a long day at school. One or two 500 milligram capsules will usually be enough to start building children's strength if they are exhausted and under stress. This amount will prevent the stress from depleting children's reserves and vitality, and negatively impacting their bodies.

At night, if your children have trouble falling asleep, 500 milligrams of ashwaganda can be taken at bedtime to help give their body the strength and stamina to wind down in the evening.

Menstrual Beginnings
When discussing adaptogenic herbs, it is important to include a significant herb used in Ayurveda to support a girl's body as she transitions through puberty to womanhood and has regular monthly menstrual cycles.

After I began my training in Ayurvedic medicine, I hosted many Ayurvedic doctors from India as they toured the United States. During their visits, we would discuss at length the differences between the conditions they would typically see in India and what they would see here in America. Invariably they would ask why so many America women have difficulties with their reproductive organs. In the U.S., a significant number of women are on hormone replacement therapy, have had a hysterectomy, or experience a wide range of menstrual difficulties. In India (as well as many other Asian countries), these conditions are rare and the doctors were shocked when they witnessed the overwhelming number of complaints American women have in this area.

The consensus among researchers and health professionals as to what may be at bottom of this American tendency is that women in the West never stop. They are asked to be a mom, run a business, exercise, raise kids, cook food, drive to soccer practices, and be a wife all at the same time. When the menstrual cycle comes around, American women don't skip a beat—they keep pushing their way through to Super-Momhood. Men could never handle the pressures and expectations that are piled on women today. It is not surprising that heart disease, which is the number-one killer in America, presently affects men and women equally. Women now share the dubious honor of succumbing to heart disease at the high rates once relegated only to men. The life we live now is too much for any human being to keep up with, but the question remains: How do we get off this speeding train?

In Ayurveda, the first two or three days of the menstrual cycle (which are the first two to three days of blood flow) are an extremely important time in the physiology of a woman's body. This is a time of physical cleansing that occurs monthly, but only in women. Men do not have a comparable cleansing process. It has been theorized that the reason why women generally live longer is because their bodies have the opportunity to cleanse and detoxify on a monthly basis. During these few days, the body's intention and focus is on moving impurities down and allowing them to flow out of the body.

But if a woman is moving full speed ahead in her life, traveling at 90 miles per hour, all the available energy in her body is detoured away from the task of releasing impurities. Over time, the overruling of this cleansing impulse can lead to an imbalance in the natural efficiency of menstruation and the monthly cycle. Most women would agree there is a feeling of calm and introspection that is associated with the menstrual flow. Traditionally, these days of cleansing provided an opportunity for women to engage in deep silence and to connect to the source within.

After this monthly dip into the sea of consciousness, women's insight could direct the decisions of the family or tribe from a renewed connection to their source.

Today, our busy schedules and hectic lives make it difficult for women to stop and rest during the first days of menstruation. An awareness and appreciation of the body's natural tendency to go within can make all the difference between an experience that is comfortable and flows with nature's cycles and one that painfully fights against the current. Whenever possible, schedule intense travel and activity around the monthly cycle. Try not to run a marathon on those days (literally or figuratively). Female athletes regularly report that if they compete on the first few days of their cycle they notice a significant drop in performance.

> Menstruation was never a sign of weakness, but a time of inner power and introspection.

Teaching girls about supporting their bodies through their menstrual cycle should be done so they can flow with the fluctuations of their cycle, rather than fight against them. Girls who are going through puberty can learn to embrace their cycles. This teaching can be done through their mothers' positive examples, presenting the cycle not as a "curse," but as a gift or time of introspection. It is important to educate girls to support the natural process of their bodies, appropriately scheduling the activities of the month and using herbs to balance both their individual body and body-type. If this transition is consciously supported, our coming generations, with any luck, will avoid the negative symptoms that afflict so many American women today.

Herbs can support and strengthen women's bodies in the transitional time of puberty as well as balance the menstrual cycle throughout their lives. It is important for the health of the body as a whole that the reproductive system organs and the menstrual cycle receive sufficient energy and strength from the body. If women and girls are not careful, it can be easy for the body to steal energy from the reproductive organs to keep the rest of the systems going at top speed. There is an Ayurvedic herb that is an adaptogen specifically for the female reproductive system; it prevents the body from going into reproductive debt, or continually losing strength and energy.

The herb is called *shatavari,* or *sitawari* (*Asparagus racemosus*). Its Ayurvedic name, translated, means "a woman with 100 husbands." It is an herb that can be taken safely throughout a woman's entire reproductive life. It can be taken from the onset of menstruation; before, during, and after pregnancy; and before, during, and after menopause.

My daughters take shatavari so that they can step out on the right foot with balanced hormonal cycles. Shatavari is able to create balance not because it is a hormonal precursor, but because it is a reproductive system tonic. It helps the body produce and gather the raw materials needed to make hormones for the menstrual cycle. It is not a precursor for hormones, nor does it stimulate hormone production. It encourages the body to support its own hormonal balance instead of depending on oral hormones to do the job.

How To Take Shatavari

The best dose for an adolescent girl is 500 milligrams two (as a preventative or supportive herb) or three (to correct an imbalance) times a day.

Teenage Acne: Balancing adolescent hormones is an important preventive measure for teenage acne. Shatavari is ideal both for balancing hormones and for reducing or preventing acne. For additional herbal support, use manjistha and neem for the prevention and treatment of teenage acne.

Check the Dryness of Your Child's Skin

Dry skin can be a sign that the inside of the body—the sinuses and intestinal tract—could also be drying out. Dryness often leads to, or is indicative of, constipation or other problems with elimination; so when the skin is dry, check the elimination habits as described earlier in this chapter and in Chapter 4. If the skin is dry, the body is not sufficiently hydrated. Be sure to follow proper hydration habits as described in Chapter 5.

The skin is not only a crucial link to the lymphatic system; it is connected to the nervous system. The skin is inundated with nerve endings, and keeping the skin itself moist and lubricated protects them. If the nerve endings on the surface of the skin are dried out and irritated they can aggravate the rest of the nervous system. A regular routine of massage helps to soothe, lubricate, and pacify the nervous system as well as bring more moisture into the tissues of the skin. In Chapter 3, I described a simple and effective daily massage technique that works very well for children with dry skin. Dry skin is more common in winter kid-types.

> Dry skin is a reflection of a body in need of hydration.

Check Your Child's Pulse

Checking the pulse is a simple way to monitor your child's level of exhaustion and susceptibility to illness without invasive testing. It is an ancient technique used in traditional medicinal systems worldwide to determine if a child is overworked, coming down with something, and in need of rest.

Step 1—Determine a Baseline

First thing in the morning, or while children are still sleeping, check their resting pulse rate. It is best to do this before they get out of bed as the day's activities will complicate the reading.

The easiest way to take your child's pulse is to hold the wrist on the thumb side of hand. Here you will find the radial artery and the radial pulse. Feel this pulse and count the beats for 30 seconds.

Multiply this number by two to obtain the pulse rate in beats per minute. It is good to do this on a regular basis to determine the average, or baseline, resting pulse rate.

Step 2—Notice the Changes

The impact of stress on your children reveals itself in their pulse. If their pulse rate changes by more than ten beats per minute above or below their average, or baseline, rate, it is an alarm bell rung by the body. This alarm alerts us to the fact that the body is working overtime. If your children's stress during this time is also excessive then it is likely that this increased pulse rate will turn into a cold or another health condition.

If the heart rate changes its rhythm by 10 beats per minute or more the body's immune system may be gearing up to fight a viral or bacterial infection. The child may be exhausted, triggering a release of degenerative stress-fighting hormones (which we know is promotes disease). Whatever the reason, the impact of stress on your children (and it could be emotional stress), is so great that it can change their pulse rate by more than 10 beats per minute above or below their average.

> If the average pulse rate increases or decreases from one day to the next by more than 10 beats per minute, it indicates that the child is under stress and in need of rest.

If you get a positive reading, carefully monitor all of the other signs and symptoms of a cold mentioned in this chapter.

Employing appropriate therapy including, in this case, a rejuvenative herb or formula like ashwaganda or chywanprash is extremely important to help rebuild a depleted nervous system.

Lisa's Story

Lisa's parents had been taking her pulse to obtain a baseline and noticed that her average heart rate first thing in the morning, or while she was sleeping, was 80 beats per minute. Lisa's heart rate may normally fluctuate between 75 and 85 beats per minute. One night, Lisa's parents noticed that she was yawning and crabby during dinner and just moved the food around on her plate. She picked fights with her younger brother, and talked back when it was time to take a bath. Lisa's parents suspected she may have been over-worked and overtired, so to check their suspicions, they took her pulse to determine if it was different from her usual baseline.

That evening Lisa's pulse was 92 beats per minute; her parents' suspicions were correct. They did not feel she was sick, or that it was necessary to keep her home from school the next day, but they limited her after-school activities for a couple of days to allow her to get some extra rest. They were vigilant in checking for the indica-tions of an upcoming cold, which she might have been vulnerable to after getting run-down. They also gave her some rejuvenative herbs. Lisa especially liked chywanprash, so she took some goop twice a day for the next few days for its adaptogenic, strength-building effect. She also took ashwaganda to settle her nervous system and allow her to catch up on some quality rest.

The vigilance of Lisa's parents paid off, as they were able to notice that Lisa was in danger of getting sick before she actually came down with something. By monitoring her levels of fatigue, checking the cold indicators described in this chapter, and admin-istrating the associated therapies, they were able to help keep Lisa on the path to perfect health.

The Power of the Pulse

I first learned the technique of monitoring health by using the pulse while I was training in India. I returned home to the three young children I had at the time: two daughters aged 6 and 4, and a 3-year-old son. When I walked in the door, my wife informed me that the girls were sick with a stomach bug, and my son looked as though he would probably start throwing up at any moment. Feeling guilty that my wife had to handle all this alone, I went upstairs to check on them. I took their pulses with the techniques I had recently learned. Just as I expected, I felt beneath my fingers that their little hearts were racing.

In Ayurveda, there is more to feeling the pulse than merely making an assessment. The second part of the technique I studied includes holding the wrist for an extended period of time to restore balance to the pulse—through restoring balance the person can get well. This was the perfect time to try it. A cure would mean my wife would get her first uninterrupted night's sleep in four nights.

I started taking my children's pulses and after gently holding each child's pulse for about ten minutes, their pulse rates slowed dramatically. Their pulses not only slowed down but became very solid and stable compared to the racing, feeble pulses they had exhibited just moments before.

Throughout this experiment the kids were asleep, and they stayed asleep. That night, surprisingly, they all slept soundly. My wife was flabbergasted. She had been watching one daughter throw up for three days. The next morning, their fevers had broken, they were all perfectly fine, and we were able to share a healthy play day.

> By touching the pulse, you are touching and potentially balancing the body—accessing the entire physical body through the pumping of the heart, the mind via the emotions stored in the heart, and the spirit through its connection to the sacred heart.

In Ayurveda the pulse is a reflection of the heart, which pumps blood into every organ every two minutes. The heart houses the emotions which we protect at all costs, and it is also recognized as the spiritual or sacred heart. In Ayurveda, as well as in China, Greece, and Egypt, the pulse was the primary diagnostic tool. It is said that the art of pulse-taking is both a diagnosis and a cure all wrapped up in the few minutes of taking the pulse.

Ayurveda traditionally recommends massaging yourself and your children every day. Kids who are touched feel nourished and loved and tend to be more stable and balanced compared to kids in isolated non-loving environments. The power of healing hands may promise to be the science of the future.

How this holding of the pulse could actually cure my children is not yet clear. It may have been coincidence, but just because we do not have technology to measure subtle energy of the body does not mean it doesn't exist. Acupuncture, for instance, has no scientific explanation, yet it has been proven to be effective in hundreds of studies. I believe that science is embarking on the understanding of the spontaneous human healing system—so far unexplainable—but it may soon be the fascination of once-dubious Western medicine.

Pools, Airplanes, and Back-to-School Days

Swimming Pools
Water can involve risky business. Swimming in a pool is refreshing in the heat of summer, but you must be on guard if your child is going to an indoor pool party in January. Kids can get chilled after they come out of a warm pool, still wet, into the cold winter air. The immune system becomes compromised when the body's core temperature drops as muscle tighten and the lymph becomes boggy opening the door for an infection to walk in.

To mitigate this potential cold-causing situation, there are fortunately several herbs which can be given including: trikatu, turmeric, chywanprash, and echinacea.

Flying
Airplanes are a threat to the body's defenses because of recycled air and the quick and rapid change of climates experienced when traveling. If, for example, you come home to Iowa after spending two weeks in Hawaii in January, you will be subject to catching a cold. This re-entry situation mimics a change of seasons.

To avoid a post-vacation cold, have your children take herbs during transitional times to support their digestion and elimination. Trifala and trikatu are both excellent for this type of support. Chywanprash and tumeric can be taken as preventive measures.

Back to School
Many parents dread the "back-to-school days" because they can really mean: "kids-home-sick days." It is a time of year when the

weather getting colder and children are coming in contact with lots of other children, exposing them to a higher concentration of cold-causing bugs. Back-to-school time comes during a change of seasons when there is already a higher risk of the mucous membranes losing their delicate balance of not-too-wet and not-too-dry. When kids go back to school there are many precautions parents can take to keep their kids healthy.

Here is a short list to review some of the suggestions that I have covered throughout the book:

- Encourage kids to go to bed early—this can be hard when it is still light at nine o'clock.
- No late, cheesy dinners or ice cream desserts.
- Eat lots of end-of-summer fruits.
- Have kids take trifala if they are constipated; watch their elimination carefully.
- Have a spoonful of chywanprash once a day for prevention.
- Have turmeric ready to give at the first hint of a runny nose.
- Keep kids hydrated.

A Cold Is Upon Us

Your child might come home from school with a fever and a sore throat. What do you do? Don't panic!

There are certain herbs that I use over and over again for these types of situations.

Echinacea is very effective if you catch the cold early enough and give it at the right dosage.

Taking lots of chywanprash is effective in the early stage of a cold. Take up to 6 teaspoons three to four times a day to knock out the cold.

Once the cold has established roots, probably the most effective remedy to fight it is turmeric. Take 1 teaspoon every one to two hours between three to seven days to fight almost any cold.

Chapter 10

Secret 9—The Lazy Susan

With six children in our house to keep healthy, I have devised a system I call the "Lazy Susan," which has become an invaluable tool when it comes to accomplishing this seemingly impossible task. The Lazy Susan that I use in my home is exactly that: a round turntable housing the most important herbal and natural supplements that I dole out to my kids on a daily basis.

In a busy house like ours, if you have to go through the effort of getting up and going over to the cupboard to pull out the supplements of the day, which may vary from kid to kid, chances are it will only happen occasionally. The Lazy Susan sits on our kitchen table and every morning I spin the wheel to see what to give my children before they go off to school. What I give them is not the same each day; it changes with the seasons, their stress levels, their current health status, and what I find in my morning inspection.

What I pull off the Lazy Susan may be as simple as a kid's multi-vitamin, if all is well and they are presently healthy. If they have eaten a heavy, cheesy dinner the night before, I may offer a digestive aid like trikatu or ginger with honey. If they have been up late with homework and are tired from their many activities at school, I will give them an adaptogen. Adaptogens are herbs (discussed in Chapter 9) that help the body cope with stress while strengthening the immune system.

If they are coming down with the sniffles, I might give them a spicy herb like ginger or turmeric with honey to break up mucus and heal the sinuses. At the beginning and end of each season, when kids are particularly susceptible to colds and the flu, I usually give them a supplement that mimics the medicinal herbs wild-crafted or harvested at that time of year.

For example:

- In the winter, I give them ashwaganda. It is a warm, heavy root harvested in the fall for winter eating. It rebuilds the nervous system during the long winter's rest.
- In the spring, I increase their intake of green vegetables. I may also use herbs and foods that are rich in green material and supplement them with two or three alfalfa tablets (we call it hay) to ensure that their intake of chlorophyll-rich foods is adequate. I also give them a tablespoon of mint-chlorophyll (available at any natural grocery) to increase their intake of green-based vegetables. Spring greens act as fertilizers for the good flora and bacterial growth of the intestinal tract.
- In the summer, cooling herbs like neem and manjistha are great choices to clean the blood, purify the skin, treat teenage acne, and improve circulatory function.

> The daily use of the Lazy Susan is all about prevention and preparation. Dealing with the effects of stress on a child is crucial to illness prevention and preparation for the future. We know that excessive stress, or the inability to cope with it, is responsible for 80% of disease and is the most significant cause of a compromised immune system. The negative impact of stress on your child is sometimes hidden. In this chapter, you will learn how to identify the signs of stress before any impact on your child's health becomes noticeable.

My goal in this chapter is to put everything together so parents have an easy-to-use guide to for how and when to use each herb. The herbs are described in more detail in previous chapters,

> If you do nothing more than follow the protocol in this chapter you will find that raising even a large family like ours is relatively simple.

but here I will review exactly how and when I use each herb with my family and my patients.

I have discussed how to discover who your children are and how to monitor them on a daily basis. I hope you are getting the idea of what to look for in order to pick up on the early warning signs of a cold-in-the-making. By noticing the signs of impending danger and having an awareness of the different seasonal food and herb choices, you be well equipped to prepare your children to combat the upcoming cold, flu, and allergy seasons.

By following the tips in this book, you will be able to anticipate and prevent seasonal vulnerabilities to illnesses three to six months before they occur. Colds that typically hit in January will have been prevented in the previous September or October. Using the preventive tools suggested in this book will soon greatly reduce the number of colds your children succumb to. And when they do come down with something, it will be a mild two- to three-day episode rather than something more severe.

Monitoring your children and increasing your awareness of their health will help them become more knowledgeable themselves of what to do to stay healthy. After all, kids don't like being sick. You will soon hear your children asking for the supplement or herb of the day off the Lazy Susan.

It was not that long ago that much of what we today call folk medicine, old wives' tales, or grandma's remedies were a part of mainstream knowledge and culture. Certain health protocols were passed down from grandmother to mother to

> Once you instill self-awareness in your children, they will know what their bodies need for the rest of their lives.

daughter, and were so ingrained in the daily routine that they were thought of as common sense. Mothers knew exactly what to do for their children, both preventively and when they got sick. Most of this simple and logical information has been forgotten and replaced with the modern approach to health care, which can be an important life-saving and valuable tool available to parents, but is limited in that it waits for an illness to take hold and become virulent before it gets treated. We have to remember that the tools of modern medicine are not the *only* tools available for parents.

Doctors of Ayurveda were traditionally paid only when all their patients were healthy. Thus, if someone became sick, the physicians were highly motivated to restore them to good health so they would get paid. Consequently, Ayurvedic doctors emphasized preventive treatments in their repertoire of skills. They monitored their patients in an especially careful manner during times of seasonal vulnerabilities, and encouraged the prevention of illnesses months before they might possibly occur.

Unfortunately, our society's health care system is not motivated to restore and maintain good health. Parents, on the other hand, are usually highly motivated to keep their children healthy. Like the ancient doctors, parents will have the best success keeping their children from getting sick by treating them preventively while they are healthy.

Secret Nine: The ninth secret is simply to follow the straightforward health care protocols that explain how and when to use these herbal preparations in the same way parents have done throughout the 5,000-year-old tradition of Ayurvedic medicine.

Aren't Herbs Dangerous?

When I worked for the New Jersey Nets, I found that many of the athletes I worked with were concerned about herbs and were reluctant to take them because of the negative experiences other athletes had had. There have been many articles and news reports about athletes having serious and even fatal reactions to certain herbal preparations. Athletes are not the only people who have had these reactions. Some herbal preparations can have very strong, often negative, effects. Some of these include products that are labeled "herbal fen-phen" or preparations with ephedra, guarana, yerba maté, hormones like DHEA and melatonin, or growth hormones and growth hormone precursors with concentrated amino acids. Herbs labeled as weight-loss aids or performance-enhancers can cause serious problems such as rapid heartbeat or cardiac irregularities. As a result of these reports, many people are under the assumption that all herbs are potentially dangerous.

It is true that herbs can have very powerful effects on the human body, especially those that stimulate or sedate, they are usually given in a concentrated extract form that exists only in a laboratory and not in nature. If someone is tired or depressed they are often prescribed an herb that is a stimulant. If someone is anxious, hyperactive, or has insomnia they are prescribed a sedative herb. People who use herbs this way might as well be taking drugs, because they're just masking symptoms. This is allopathic medicine's attempt to prescribe a "natural" substitute for a pharmaceutical concoction—but using a concentrated extract of the active ingredient of an herb is far from natural. Herbs, when examined from a traditional point of view, were never intended to be used to treat symptoms in this way. In fact, any herb that would overrule the body's ability to perform an action on its own was not typically recommended in traditional Ayurvedic medicine.

I am extremely surprised by how casually doctors who use natural medicines—nutritionists, naturopaths, and chiropractors—prescribe things like plant-based or natural hormones, growth hormone precursors, laxatives, stimulants, sedatives, and digestive enzymes. All of these often make up the bulk of a nutritionally based practice and they are all designed to perform a task or do a job *for* the body,

> Stimulants, sedatives, laxatives, or herbs that manipulate the body are not used in my practice and are definitely not recommended in this book.

often leaving the body less able to do the job itself.

For example, if a woman were prescribed hormone replacement therapy, then the presence of these hormones in the body would tell the body not to bother making its own hormones because it is already getting a free supply. The body's endocrine, or hormonal, system regulates the amount of hormones produced through feedback mechanisms: when the hormone is present in the body in the appropriate amount, further production of the hormone is turned off. If the hormone is taken continually, the body repeatedly receives the message that it doesn't need to make the hormone at all. The most logical first approach to a hormone imbalance is to use herbs or substances that stimulate the body to restore its ability to make its own hormones naturally; this is typically done with botanical hormonal precursors—an approach that has been used by Ayurvedic medicine for thousands of years.

> We have become conditioned to think it is okay to just get rid of symptoms at any cost. Antibiotics, laxatives, or stimulants like Ritalin very effectively eradicate symptoms but may quietly drive the cause of the condition deeper into your child's body. Such treatments definitely have their place. But by using them as a first round of therapy, we could be turning a simple imbalance that is easy to treat naturally into a difficult-to-treat chronic condition in the years to come.

Instead of giving your child a synthetic drug with numerous side effects, it makes sense to give a more natural supplement that allows the body to repair itself, or if that fails, give one that has a similar action to the drug, but without the side effects. In Ayurveda, the first approach to health care is to support the body's ability to heal itself. I offer herbal suggestions to support your children's ability to maintain balance, a strong immunity, a patent lymphatic circulatory system, and optimal blood supply to each and every cell of the body.

If a problem arises in a child, the approach that Ayurveda suggests is to delve to the root of the condition rather than simply treat the symptoms. If, for example, a child becomes constipated, instead of using harsh laxatives, which irritate the intestinal wall and create a dependency, Ayurveda suggests treating the cause of the condition by supporting the child's nervous system during its exposure to excessive stress, healing the intestinal mucosa, and tonifying the muscles of the large intestine in order to restore normal function. This approach is so simple and so direct, yet our culture is still fascinated with the instant results of symptomatic suppression.

> Don't be fooled! Just because something is natural—an herbal product, a dietary supplement, or sold in a health-food store—doesn't mean it's safe or effective. Many of these products are habit-forming, create dependencies, reduce the body's own ability to restore normal function, have unwanted side effects, and in many cases make the cause of the condition worse.

The herbs I suggest in this book have been tested over thousands of years as a part of Ayurvedic medicine. Most of the herbs that I use in my practice are actually foods and spices, many of which were a part of the American diet less than a hundred years ago. These substances are natural and are easily absorbed, assimilated, and digested like foods, not drugs. Because these herbs are more food than drug, and because the whole herb contains all of the chemicals in the plant, not just one or two isolated compounds, the body can absorb the components of the herbal food it needs for the situation at hand. If the body does not require a specific herbal constituent, it is easily passed through the body as waste.

Herbs can also be extracted, at which point they are called herbal extracts. These isolate one active chemical of the plant and concentrate it into a pill or liquid. An intensified dose of the active ingredient is then given. I feel that when you take a single chemical out of a plant and administer it separately from the whole plant, it then becomes a drug rather than an herbal medicine.

Any plant contains a complex spectrum of chemical constituents that interact with each other in the body, helping to balance the effect of the plant, thus making it safer to take a whole herb rather than a pure concentrated extract. There are some extracts, however, that concentrate the entire plant, including all of its constituents. In most cases this is an ideal situation: the supplement is less intense, the dose of the active chemicals is milder, and the effects are greater without producing harmful side effects.

Stimulants, sedatives, and laxatives that are extracts of a single active ingredient can be dangerous. Most of the herbal formulations that have caused harm to athletes were stimulants designed to improve performance or to treat colds. Such stimulants often interact with seemingly harmless over-the-counter medications with potentially catastrophic consequences. These herbs—marketed as cure-alls that provide instant energy, promise bigger muscles, and say that your cold will be gone in a day—should be avoided.

Remember: if it sounds too good to be true, it probably is.

There is a natural progression that should be followed when using any intervention, whether herbal or pharmaceutical. All treatments exist for a reason and have their place, but should only be used when appropriate. If someone needs medical intervention because of an illness or imbalance, it makes sense to use the gentlest treatment first, usually one that supports the body's own ability to heal itself and treats the cause of the condition. If these herbs do not do the trick, then the next logical approach is to take a stronger symptom-based approach: a natural supplement or a more natural herbal form of a drug. If that fails, a Western pharmaceutical medication should be taken with the knowledge that this strong, concentrated medication is the last resort. Pharmaceutical drugs save lives and should be taken when necessary.

In our culture we use the term alternative medicine to describe the alternative to modern Western drugs. This is a backward and illogical approach to health care. As described above, pharmaceutical drugs, often stronger than natural herbs and supplements, should be the alternative when more natural and gentler substances are not effective in the individual circumstance. Western medicinal substances should not be considered the enemy; they should have their appropriate place as part of a more logical protocol—preferably a protocol that motivates doctors and parents to maintain their children's health and treat the cause of the condition the way it has been done since ancient times.

What About Vitamins?
It wasn't long ago that we and our children ingested vitamins and minerals in our foods in the quantities necessary to maintain optimal health, growth, and development. Even today, very large vegetarian animals like elephants, deer, elk, and moose seem to do quite well without the aid of multivitamin and mineral supplements. So why is it that we now being told to supplement our diets with vitamins? An article published in the *Journal of the American Medical Association (JAMA)* in 2002 advises that all adults take at least one multivitamin pill each day. Twenty years ago the same journal published a comprehensive review of vitamins that reported that the average person shouldn't take multivitamins because they were a waste of time and money.

Things have changed in the last 20 years. Clearly, we are under more stress than ever before. Our diets are lacking in adequate fresh fruits and vegetables, and the foods harvested today are deficient in the vitamins, minerals, and trace elements that were common in the soils 50 years ago. The 2002 *JAMA* article was from a recent Harvard University study—just one example of the research attention and approval that vitamins are receiving today versus the negative press they received only 20 years ago.

In a 2002 USDA study, the meals of 20,000 people were tested over a period of three days for the 10 most essential nutrients. Amazingly, not one meal—not one person's meal—contained the minimum requirements, according to the Recommended Daily Allowance (RDA). Other studies also reveal that something is missing in our diets. Dr. Robert Fletcher of Harvard University reported that almost 80% of Americans do not eat the minimum suggested amount of five servings of fruits and vegetables each day needed to provide the body with sufficient nutrients.

We are not meeting even the *suggested* Recommended Daily or Dietary Allowance of nutrients in our food, but alarmingly, these values may be too low. The RDA levels were set at the minimum amounts of the nutrients needed to *avoid deficiencies*. There is new and compelling evidence that the minimum amount of a nutrient needed to avoid a deficiency is much less than the actual amount of the nutrient needed to maintain good health. According to Dr. Fletcher, even people who eat five daily servings of fruits and vegetables may not be taking in high enough levels of all the vitamins necessary for optimal health.

The general consensus explaining the reason why the RDAs are too low is multifold. Not only were they initially set at low levels, but the stress that American adults and children are subjected to has been increasing over time. The body demands higher-quality nutrition to cope with the assault of constant stress. Additionally, the excessive amounts of empty calories, sugars, and refined flours, along with environmental pollutants and the aforementioned stress can deplete B-vitamins and nutrients from the body. How foods are stored also affects their vitamin content. Many vitamins, such as Vitamin C, degrade over time, and are found in smaller quantities in those foods that have been transported over long distances than in those foods that have been bought and consumed near where they were grown. And, finally, the soils of today are clearly deficient in the minerals and trace elements necessary to provide high-quality and nutritious foods.

As early as 1936, scientific authorities and the U.S. government registered concern about the nutritional quality of the food being grown in American soil. The now-famous Senate Document 264, written and presented by Rex Beach, stated that 99% of American people are deficient in "mineral salts" important in the diet. The report stated that "No man of today [this is in 1936!] can eat enough fruits and vegetables to supply his stomach with the mineral salts he requires for perfect health, because his stomach isn't big enough to hold them!" The report continued: "Laboratory tests prove that the fruits, the vegetables, the grains, the eggs, and even the milk and the meats of today are not what they were a few generations ago." The report stated that not all carrots are created equal, and not all carrots contain what they are supposed to contain. If these were concerns nearly a hundred years ago, before the widespread use of soil-disrupting chemical fertilizers and the prevalence of factory-farming mono-crop cultivation rather than soil-building crop rotation, they are even of more concern today. The change in agricultural practices and the further depletion of the soil has left us short of the nutrients we need for health.

With the deficiencies in today's soils—combined with both the highly processed, nutrient-deficient foods that make up most of the American diet and with rising stress levels—it is amazing that children today do as well as they do. Another report in the *American Journal of Public Health* stated that only 9% of Americans eat the recommended servings of fruits and vegetables per day, and on an average day 45% of Americans do not eat any fruits or drink any fruit juice, and 22% do not eat any vegetables. These results make the case for taking vitamin supplements much more compelling.

I think at this point it is clear to most parents that both children and adults need some type of nutritional supplementation. According to many studies, it seems that no matter how well you feed your family, they will come up short somewhere on the nutritional stick. So the questions remain: What type of vitamins should you buy for your family? How do you know if the vitamin is of good quality and is being absorbed into the bloodstream and cells so it can be properly utilized? These are questions that, unfortunately, are often not asked. If we assume that all vitamin and mineral supplements are created equal, we may be in for a surprise.

According to a 1992 study by Dr. Gsell-Schleettwein entitled: "Outcome of Nutritional Intervention," 97% of Americans have some sort of nutritional (vitamin or mineral) deficiency. Yet, according to the previously mentioned study published in *JAMA,* 33% of Americans are taking multivitamins as a part of their diet. If 97% of the American population has a nutritional deficiency, and 33% of Americans are taking multivitamins regularly, then we can conclude that the majority of the vitamins people are taking are not work-ing. Only a very low 3% of Americans have adequate nutrition and are deficiency-free.

> How do you know if the vitamins you are offering your children are being absorbed and assimilated efficiently? The best way to find out is to contact your vitamin company and ask it for its absorption rates for the vitamins and minerals in its product. If you do this, many companies will tell you that they have 100% absorption rates. I would then suggest you ask the company to fax you a copy of the nutritional assay or absorption rate study. I have done this and have yet to receive a single study from any company.

The bottom line is that most companies make claims about absorption rates based on the theory or concept of how the vitamins and minerals are delivered to the cells. In my research, I have not been able to find definite information in this area. According to one independent researcher I spoke with, most vitamin and mineral products absorb at surprisingly low levels. Minerals, which are the hardest substances for the body to deliver to the cells, are absorbed in the ranges of 10% to 50% of what is taken into the body. What is not delivered to the cells is being eliminated, processed, or stored in the deep tissues of the body.

The problem with taking vitamins and minerals that do not absorb completely is that the body is then forced to detoxify and remove these hard-to-digest substances through the eliminative channels. Unfortunately, not all of the unprocessed and unabsorbed vitamins and minerals are fully eliminated from the body. Many of these undigested substances can be stored in the tissues, building up as a form of *ama,* or toxic material, that was mentioned in Chapter 4. This is something that parents should be aware of, as rec-ommendations to take vitamins on a daily basis are now coming from even conservative sources like the *Journal of the American Medical Association.*

Not all vitamins and minerals are created equal. The best rec-ommendation I can make is to take a vitamin supplement that is derived from plant extracts. Synthetic vitamins claim to be bio-identical to natural vitamins and to function just as well in the body as the naturally occurring vitamins in fruits and vegetables. There are, however, trace elements and minerals that co-occur with natural vitamins and minerals. These are recognized by the body as a food source and, as a result, are well-absorbed by the deep tissues. Synthetic vitamins, while they may be broken down in the digestive system, are in fact not bio-identical at the most basic level; they do not have the co-occurring trace elements and therefore are not absorbed as easily into the deep tissues. For example, in the case of Vitamin A, retinol (the synthetic version of Vitamin A), has been shown to increase the risk of hip fractures and loss of bone density.

An interesting study using essential oils examined the difference between synthetic/bio-identical oils and biological material originating from plants. The study measured the effects of the scented oils on brain-wave wave functioning, comparing a source from actual plant biological material with oil that was synthetic but seemingly bio-identical. Rose oil absolute, which is made exclusively from rose petals, was compared to synthetic rose oil that was chemically bio-identical. When the synthetic rose oil was inhaled, there was no effect on, or change in, brain-wave wave function. But when the rose absolute was inhaled, the brain waves dramatically shifted.

The conclusion of this study indicated that the sense of smell directed to the brain has an inhibitory mechanism that is still not completely understood. The body allowed the absolute rose to penetrate the limbic system—the part of the brain that affects emotions and the place where the sense of smell is first directed. The rose absolute caused a change in brain waves. On the other hand, the body did not recognize the so-called bio-identical, synthetic rose oil as natural, so its entry into the limbic system was inhibited, and it was unable to affect brain-wave wave function.

We do not know enough about the effect of synthetic vitamins on the body, whether they have a positive, negative or neutral effect, so play it safe and use natural, plant-based products. There is still

Making sure your children eat plenty of servings of fruits, vegetables, nuts, seeds, and whole grains is step one in multimineral and multivitamin supplementation.

much to be studied, learned, and understood about the absorption, utilization, and quality of vitamins and minerals. The one thing we know for certain is that humans are designed to absorb and assimilate their vitamins and minerals from foods like fruits and vegetables. If the source of the vitamins and minerals is plant-based, then the chances of absorption are significantly greater.

Step two is to purchase a vitamin and mineral supplement from a reputable company that is composed of plant-sourced ingredients.

It is probably not necessary, if the nutritional base provided by your children's diet is good, to give them multivitamin and mineral supplements each and every day. If you are giving them a daily dose of some type of preventive herbs like chywanprash (see Chapter 9), you can give the vitamin supplement somewhere between three and six days a week, rather than every day.

Parental Tip: Don't buy the cheapest chewable vitamins at the grocery store and expect them to be absorbed and utilized efficiently by the body.

Buy your vitamins from a reputable health-food store, health care practitioner, or vitamin company that you know and trust. The best vitamin company is one that makes their absorption rates available. I am continually investigating companies that offer the highest absorption rates available. For more information on this subject, you can e-mail me at: info@lifespa.com. I will be able to give you the most current information I have on absorption rates and vitamins.

You can also contact the National Nutritional Foods Association at 800.966.6632, or www.nnfa.org. The NNFA is an organization that certifies nutritional companies who adhere to "good manufacturing processes." This means the products are what they say they are, the products are tracked with lot numbers, and the manufacturing plants are clean. The United States Pharmacopoeia, www.usp-dsvp.org, checks and runs tests on products to ensure that product labels and their ingredients are consistent. Both of these nonprofit organizations publish a list of the products they have tested.

There are, I am sure, many products not tested by these organizations that are of high quality. Although these lists can be helpful, they are not comprehensive enough to pass judgment on all nutritional products.

Lazy Susan

The Lazy Susan I described at the beginning of this chapter is where I keep the nutritional products I use most often in my quest for optimal health for my family. The following list contains my Lazy Susan supplements ranked in general order of frequency of use. I state the herb, what chapter you can find more information, including dosage, and what its most common therapeutical use is. Then, I provide lists detailing the kid-type and seasonal effects of the herbs. I also include a list of common conditions and the herbs used for treatment and prevention as a cross-reference. To choose an herb for your children, first find the herb that suits their symptoms and then check it against the kid-type and seasonal list.

Lazy Susan Herbs

Primary List
Trikatu—See Chapters 4 and 7

- Late-night snacks or heavy dinners
- Eating a new diet while traveling
- Illness prevention during seasonal changes
- While traveling and to use for post-vacation reentry to home climate
- First sign of a runny nose
- Allergies or allergy season
- Sinus infections
- Sore throats

Trifala—See Chapter 4
- Heavy dinners
- Prevention of travel constipation
- First sign of a cold: circles under the eyes
- Sluggish elimination
- Constipation
- Gentle intestinal cleanse
- Multimineral and multivitamin supplements (see Chapter 10)
- Prevention and maintenance three to six times per week

Turmeric—See Chapters 3 and 4
- Runny nose
- Cold or flu
- Diarrhea
- Allergies
- Any type of inflammation
- Cough
- Skin disorder or rash
- Indigestion

Ashwaganda—See Chapter 9
- Fatigue
- Stress
- Compromised immune system
- Excessive exercise or schoolwork
- Undesired weight loss
- Memory improver and strengthener

Bacopa—See Chapter 12
- Depression
- Energy
- Attention Deficit
- Improves memory

Chywanprash—See Chapter 9
- Daily nutrition
- Immune system strengthener
- First sign of a cold

- Feeling of being run down
- Vitamin C supplement
- Instant energy or snack

Sitopladi—See Chapter 3
- Lung congestion
- Asthma or breathing difficulties
- Cough, dry or productive
- Bronchitis

Sitopladi-Turmeric Mix—See Chapter 3
- Cough
- Breathing difficulties
- Infection, cold or flu

Sitopladi-Turmeric-Trikatu Mix—See Chapters 3 and 4
- Upper sinus infection
- Cough
- Cold and/or flu
- Inflamed sinuses with productive mucus

Secondary List

Gymnema—See Chapter 6
- Sugar cravings
- Hypoglycemia, mood changes
- Low afternoon energy

Chewable Colostrum—See Chapter 8
- Immune system builder
- Heals dry and irritated mucous membranes

Echinacea—See Chapter 9
- Initial sign of a cold
- Strengthens immune system and moves stagnant lymph

Fenugreek—See Chapter 4
- Slow digestion
- Bloating

- Constipation

Cumin-Ginger Tea—See Chapter 4
- Gas and/or bloating

Hing (Asafoetida)—See Chapter 4
- Gas
- Bloating
- Intestinal cramping
- Constipation
- Tummyache

Fennel-Cumin-Hing—See Chapter 4
- Tummyache

Ginger Digestive Aids—See Chapter 4
- Late-night heavy dinners
- Indigestion

Trifala and Bilva—See Chapter 4
- Diarrhea

Castor Oil (Castor Oil Cookie Recipe)—See Chapter 4
- Constipation

Shatavari (sitawari)—See Chapter 9
- Helps to prepare adolescent girls for menstruation

Ear Oil—See Chapter 9
- Once every two to four weeks in the winter for prevention
- Sinus infection
- Cold or flu
- Earache

Fennel-Coriander Tea—See Chapter 4
- Stomach acidity
- Excess heat

Neem—See Chapter 4
- Skin Rashes (See Chapter 4)

- Fever
- Acne

Manjistha—See Chapters 3 and 4
- Lymphatic stagnation
- Skin rashes, eczema
- Swollen glands
- Puffy eyes
- Itchy skin, worse with exercise
- Fatigue
- Acne
- Allergies

Essential Oils—See Chapter 10

The following items obviously don't live on the Lazy Susan, but are part of our daily regimen:

Digestion and Cold Soup—See Chapter 4
- Cold or flu
- Recovery from stomach problems
- poor digestion

Daily Massage—See Chapter 3
- Dry Skin
- Stress
- Improves lymph drainage
- Protection during cold season
- Winter prevention

Hydration—See Chapter 5
- Colds
- Indigestion
- Allergies, asthma
- Prevention of almost everything

Herbs That Balance Each Kid-Type and Season

My list of Lazy Susan herbs is classified by their effect on the kid-type and the season. This information will help you avoid administering herbs that could potentially aggravate your child's kid-type.

For example, if your child has a rash, you may think of neem, which is indicated for rashes. But if your child has irritated eczema, and he or she is a winter kid-type, *and* this complaint is during the winter season, the cooling property of neem may aggravate the child's already dry nature and condition.

But if your child is a summer kid-type and complains of a red, inflamed rash in August, neem may be just the herb to clear it up. The cool nature of neem will chill the inflammation, bringing relief to the symptoms and addressing the cause of the problem.

> The following list will help a parent cross-reference the herbs for their child's kid-type and specific imbalance. First find the herb or herbs that suit your child's needs and then check them against this list for kid-type and seasonal indications.

 Note: Many herbs are suited for more than one kid-type and season. Some formulas are very well balanced and effective for all types and all seasons.

Herbal remedies that balance winter, or Vata

- Trikatu
- Trifala
- Ashwaganda
- Chywanprash
- Bacopa
- Echinacea
- Sitopladi
- Daily oil massage
- Tummyache formula (fennel, cumin, hing)
- Gas Bloating Formula (cumin-ginger tea)

- Turmeric: small amounts
- Shatavari (Sitawari)
- Fennel-coriander tea
- Colostrum
- Hing
- Digestion and cold soup
- Ear oil
- Fenugreek
- Ginger digestive aids
- Castor oil
- Grapefruit seed extract

Herbal remedies that balance summer, or Pitta

- Neem
- Manjistha
- Fennel-coriander tea
- Tummyache formula (fennel, cumin,hing)
- Shatavari (Sitawari)
- Echinacea
- Sitopladi
- Trifala
- Colostrum
- Digestion and cold soup
- Daily oil massage
- Ear oil
- Hing (small quantities)
- Trifala and Bilva
- Gymnema
- Chywanprash

Herbal remedies that balance spring, or Kapha

- Fenugreek
- Gymnena
- Sitopladi
- Trifala

- Tummyache formula (fennel, cumin, hing)
- Daily oil massage
- Colostrum
- Bacopa
- Digestion and cold soup
- Ear oil
- Turmeric
- Chywanprash
- Hing
- Echinacea
- Manjistha
- Neem
- Fennel-coriander tea
- Ashwaganda
- Trikatu
- Ginger digestive aids
- Gas and bloating formula (cumin-ginger tea)

Lazy Susan Conditions and Treatments

Acne
Neem—See Chapter 4
Manjistha—See Chapters 3 and 4

Allergies
Trifala—See Chapter 4
Turmeric—See Chapters 3 and 4
Trikatu—See Chapters 4 through 7

Asthma
Sitopladi—See Chapter 3
Colostrum—See Chapter 8
Trikatu—See Chapters 4 and 7

Attention Deficit
Bacopa—See Chapter 12

Colds
Turmeric—See Chapters 3 and 4
Sitopladi—See Chapter 3
Trikatu—See Chapter 4
Ear oil—See Chapter 9
Echinacea—See Chapter 9

Constipation
Trifala—See Chapter 4
Castor oil—See Chapter 4
Chywanprash—See Chapter 9
Fenugreek—See Chapter 4

Cough
Sitopladi—See Chapter 3
Sitopladi, Turmeric—See Chapter 3
Sitopladi, Turmeric, Trikatu—See Chapters 3 and 4

Diarrhea
Trifala with Bilva—See Chapter 4
Blackberry—See Chapter 4
Nutmeg—See Chapter 4
Pomegranate—See Chapter 4

Digestive Gas/Bloating/Tummyache
Hing—See Chapter 4
Cumin-ginger tea—See Chapter 4
Fennel, cumin, hing—See Chapter 4
Fenugreek—See Chapter 4

Fatigue
Ashwaganda—See Chapter 9
Bacopa—See Chapter 12
Chywanprash—See Chapter 9
Manjistha—See Chapters 3 and 4

Fever
Manjistha—See Chapters 3 and 4
Neem—See Chapter 4
Chywanprash—See Chapter 9
Colostrum—See Chapter 8

Hypoglycemia
Gymnema—See Chapter 6

Memory
Bacopa—See Chapter 12
Ashwaganda—See Chapter 9

Menstruation
Shatwari (Sitawari)—See Chapter 9

Rash
Neem—See Chapter 4
Manjistha—See Chapters 3 and 4
Turmeric—See Chapters 3 and 4

Sinus Infection
Echinacea—See Chapter 9
Trikatu—See Chapters 4 and 7
Ear oil—See Chapter 9
Turmeric—See Chapters 3 and 4

Slow Digestion
Fenugreek—See Chapter 4
Trifala—See Chapter 4
Castor oil—See Chapter 4
Chywanprash—See Chapter 9

Swollen Glands
Manjistha—See Chapters 3 and 4

Daily massage—See Chapter 3
Ear oil—See Chapter 9

Tummyache
Fennel, cumin, hing—See Chapter 4
Ginger digestive aids—See Chapter 4

A Word on Dosages
Suggested dosages for each herb are indicated in detail in the chapter where each herb is described (reference the index). A good general rule of thumb to use when deciding the dosage of an herb to give your children is based on their age. Take their age and divide it by 20 to give you the portion of the adult dose that should be used for the child.

> Age/20 = portion of adult dose for a child. For example, the dose of an herb for a 6-year-old child would be: 6/20 or 3/10 (30%) of a full adult dose.

In the detailed information about the herb in each chapter, I make recommendations for how to take specific herbal preparations. If kids are able to tolerate the taste of an herb mixed with honey into a paste and can eat it off a spoon with something to drink afterwards, that is the ideal Ayurvedic way to take an herb. But even though many kids will take herbs this way, others cannot stand the taste. If they find the taste unpalatable, it can make administering these herbs a torture for parents and kids alike. In this case, give them herbs in capsules, which break down quickly in the stomach to release the herb effectively.

In my home, I successfully convinced the kids to swallow capsules—even when they were only 3 or 4 years old. But, I didn't have much success convincing them logically by telling how great they would feel if they took the herb, and that they really needed it or they would have to go to the doctor. Basically, I had tried everything without success, so I bribed them. Yes, you may not think this is an acceptable way for getting your kids to do what you want, but it worked. The fact that all of our kids have been able to take capsules has saved the health of our household countless times.

I told them that if they could take this capsule then we would go to the toy store and they could get anything they wanted. This, along with a little reverse psychology—telling them that I didn't think they could do it and leaving the room a little disappointed— proved to be a big motivator. Within minutes each kid was able to swallow a capsule. You have to catch them when they are young enough not to realize what a big deal swallowing a pill is. All they hear is "Toy Store" and they swallow the pill just as easily as a spoonful of mashed potatoes or applesauce.

Essential Oils

Essential oils are the essence of plants, herbs, or flowers. An essential oil is a steam-distillation preparation of the plant that yields its most concentrated medicine. Essential oils are aromatic and effective in aromatherapy, a powerful method of using herbs by accessing the sense of smell. This is our only sense that directly accesses the limbic system—the emotional center of the brain— through the olfactory nerve. This is why when you smell a familiar scent it can instantly trigger memories or past experiences.

> The oil itself is the most powerful and medicinal part of a plant.

How To Use Essential Oils

Essential oils can be diffused in your children's rooms at night while they're sleeping or added to their daily massage oil. For massage, typically a dilution of 5% is effective. To diffuse into the night air in the bedroom, 10 or 20 drops of an essential oil in hot water is effective. Aromatherapy diffusers, which disperse oils more efficiently (especially the ones that come with programmable timers), are available in health food stores and specialty shops.

How To Use the List of Oils

The list of essential oils below are specific to balance each kid-type: winter, summer, and spring. The oils can be chosen either specifically to calm the body type of the

> The use of essential oils dates back thousands of years and it continues to be effective, popular, and scientifically verifiable.

child or for use in the season that will potentially aggravate your child's constitution. For example, if your child is a summer kid-type, then choose an oil from the summer list of essential oils.

Some oils are extremely effective for all three constitutional types. These tri-type oils are especially valuable from a mental and emotional point of view. If your child is acting out or having trouble settling down at night, select one of the tri-type oils and diffuse it in the bedroom as he or she goes to sleep.

Note: There are many excellent reference books on essential oils and aromatherapy. The oils in the following list are better described in books that specialize in the subject. When you discover which symptoms these oils treat, you can further fine-tune your selection by combining body-type information with the type of imbalance your child has. For example, there may be two or three oils that treat your child's breathing difficulty; but only one that fits your child's constitution, season, and cause of the condition.

Winter Oils

- Basil
- Fennel
- Marjoram
- Orange
- Geranium
- Bergamot
- Benzoin
- Cardamom
- Cinnamon

Summer Oils

- Sandalwood
- Lavender
- Lemon
- Ylang Ylang
- Chamomile
- Peppermint
- Fennel
- Rose
- Neroli
- Melissa (lemon balm)

Spring Oils

- Rosemary
- Eucalyptus
- Camphor
- Frankincense
- Clary sage
- Juniper
- Myrrh
- Black pepper
- Clove

Tri-type Oils

- Rose
- Jasmine
- Lavender
- Sandalwood
- Frankincense
- Melissa (lemon balm)
- Ginger
- Fennel

Chewing the Winter Fat

As we have discussed throughout this book, there are times in the year when your children are likely to be more susceptible to getting sick. One of these times is at the end of a season, when the properties of the season have built up to their most intense level, and the weather is changing and transitioning to the next season. At the end of each season we all have an increased vulnerability to catching a cold, developing allergies, or experiencing breathing difficulties such as asthma. The end of winter is a dangerous time because the dryness and cold in the environment has accumulated to its maximum level. To protect the body from the parched dryness, it is important to increase the intake of essential fatty acids in the diet.

Essential fatty acids, or EFAs, are a necessary part of our dietary intake and are different from the other oils in the diet. They are important in neurotransmitter function and the development of the myelin sheath (the protective coating around nerves), making them supportive to the nervous system. They are also essential components of the immune system, making them necessary for maintaining strong immunity. EFAs contribute to the integrity of membranes, including the skin, digestive tract, and walls of arteries and other vessels. Studies have shown that taking EFAs reduces levels of blood cholesterol in children, and as a result, they have a protective effect against heart disease later in life. EFAs have also been shown to have beneficial effects in many chronic diseases, including diabetes, arthritis, and asthma.

Because EFAs are very fragile and break down easily, it is common for children to have deficiencies in these essential nutrients. EFAs are easily damaged through exposure to air, light, high temperatures, and food processing. Most vegetable oils found in crackers, chips, cookies, and cereals are processed, and as a result have

> The body does not manufacture EFAs, so they must be taken as food or as a dietary supplement. They are most commonly available in cold-water fish, leafy green vegetables, cold-pressed vegetable oils, dried legumes, and raw nuts (especially walnuts) and seeds.

a damaging effect on the body. The hydrogenation process that is used for oils found in many types of margarine and packaged foods not only damages the essential fatty acids normally found in the oils, but actually makes them harmful to the body. It has been shown that hydrogenated vegetable oils increase cholesterol and free radicals. When oils are hydrogenated, trans-fatty acids are produced. This type of fat is thought to be even more dangerous to cardiovascular health than saturated fats and should be avoided whenever possible. Current labeling requires many foods to state the percentage of trans-fatty acids in the foods.

There are two kinds of EFAs: Omega-3 and Omega-6 oils. Omega-6 oils are commonly found in most quality, minimally processed vegetable oils. Omega-3 oils, on the other hand, are less likely to be part of a child's standard diet, and as a result many children become deficient in these important fats. Omega-3 oils are found in cold-water fish such as salmon and cod. Some other good sources of Omega-3 oils are: cod liver oil, flaxseed oil or freshly ground flax seeds, leafy green vegetables, beans, freshly ground wheat germ, and nuts (particularly walnuts). These oils are particularly fragile and unstable, so these foods must be eaten as fresh as possible. This is one of the reasons why buying food fresh and in season from your local farmer is good for your family's health.

If your children are deficient in essential fatty acids some of the symptoms they may experience include:

- chronic congestion
- chronic runny nose
- earaches
- coughs of prolonged duration
- allergies
- asthma
- skin rashes
- digestive problems

In Norway in the winter, children are required to take a daily dose of cod liver oil, typically 1 teaspoon per day. Since winter is the time of the year that the body is storing its fats, minerals, vitamins, and proteins, cod liver oil ensures that a child gets adequate amounts of Vitamin D to build healthy bones and EFAs to support a strong immune system. Flax seed oil can also be used, given during the winter months at a child's dosage of 1 teaspoon per day.

Trifala and trikatu are very effective preventive herbs to use during the transition from winter to spring.

Winter illness prevention requires a higher protein and higher fat diet (including sufficient EFAs) in the winter season with adequate sources of vitamins and minerals—the co-factors that work with EFAs to do their job of supporting the immune system.

Spring Ahead

The rainy, wet spring brings an increased susceptibility to colds and allergies as a result of excess mucus production. The best way to prevent excess mucus in the spring is to properly follow a winter diet. Remember that the body makes excess mucus in the spring to the extent that it was dried out in the winter.

> Toward the end of winter, supporting effective elimination keeps the body from becoming excessively dry and building up toxic material, or *ama*.

The austere spring harvest contains an abundance of salads, leafy green vegetables, and sprouts. Leafy greens like kale, chard, dandelion leaves, and other bitter greens like spinach are very helpful during this time of year. And local herbs like burdock, dandelion, goldenseal, and Oregon grape roots, all of which break up excess mucus, are naturally harvested and can be added to the diet.

Herbs from the Lazy Susan like turmeric, trikatu, fenugreek, chywanprash, and trifala can help remove excess mucus and strengthen digestion in order to keep your children free of colds and allergies. As mentioned earlier, adding alfalfa and chlorophyll to the diet in spring helps to strengthen the digestive system.

> The spring harvest brings with it the means by which to cleanse excess mucus from the body.

Staying Cool in the Summer

At the end of summer, the body is likely to dry out from the accumulated heat. This heat also can provoke end-of-summer allergies like hay fever and predispose the child to an excess of reactive mucus production in the winter.

Apples, pomegranates, watermelons, pears, and grapes are some of the commonly harvested fruits designed to cool the body and prevent it from becoming overly hot and dry. Give your children permission to eat more of these foods at the end of summer.

Summer kid-types also need to be shade-lovers; they should stay out of the direct summer sun, especially in the mid-afternoon. By nature, they are not usually inclined to sunbathe. In the summer, parents should encourage exercise in the morning or early evening rather than under the heat of the midday sun. Because the sun is in the sky more of the day in this season, parents can extend summer bedtimes and let the kids stay up later.

Some of the very cooling herbs like neem and manjistha can be taken preventively at this time of year. At the end of the summer, adding trifala and chywanprash to the diet for a couple of weeks can provide extremely effective cold protection in the transitional time and throughout the upcoming months.

Check the 3-Season Grocery Chart in Chapter 7 for a complete list of the seasonal foods appropriate for each time of year.

The key for summer health is to serve meals filled with the naturally available cooling foods and fruits.

Chapter 11

Secret 10—Health Is Just
a Breath Away

Ayurveda is one of the many traditional medical systems that emphasize breathing through the nose and actively cultivate this ability. Babies naturally breathe primarily through their noses, but as kids get older, they more often breathe through their mouths. In traditional medical systems and cultures that favor nasal breathing, parents train their children to continue to breathe through their noses. If parents see children sleeping on their back with their mouths wide open, they turn them on their side, close their mouths, and pinch their lips to keep them nasal breathing. The practice of nasal breathing has been cultivated for thousands of years because many tribal peoples discovered that nasal-breathing kids caught fewer colds. It is also understood that nasal breathing creates a stronger nervous system and develops a sharper intellect. Numerous studies have been conducted by the Indian military comparing nasal-breathing troops to mouth-breathing troops. The mouth-breathing troops succumbed to more colds and viral infections than their healthy nasal-breathing counterparts.

The skill of nasal breathing has been taught by parents throughout history the way we teach our children to swim. It is valued not only for its health and physical performance benefits, but also for the access it provides to the development of our full mental and spiritual potential. Ayurveda, the science of life, emphasizes the connection between body, mind, and spirit and was originally designed to prepare the body to support its spiritual process.

> Nasal breathing is key to the development of a child's nervous system and for achieving a successful spiritual life. The breath opens the doors of the central nervous system and brain so that the subtle energy of the body can be felt.

When I wrote my first book, *Body, Mind, and Sport,* in 1992, I was ridiculed when I introduced the concept of nasal breathing during exercise. According to conventional belief at the time, there was no difference between breathing through the mouth and breathing through the nose. But no one knew for certain, since Western physiology textbooks clearly stated that the complete functions of the respiratory tract were not yet understood. (Even today, they are not fully understood.) Our lungs have a total of five lobes. The majority of people breathe only into the two upper lobes, leaving most of their lung space dormant—what is called "dead air space." When I began my investigations into breathing and exercise, one question I had was: "If we have five lobes in our lungs, why aren't they all functional?"

The right way to breathe was historically passed from mother to daughter and father to son as a natural part of raising a child. Parents simply corrected their children's breathing and reset their sleeping position if they were mouth breathing at night. During waking hours, when children were spending time with their parents in activities like hiking into the forest, gathering food for the family or fresh leaves for the cows, they would naturally imitate their parents' breathing style—through the nose. This is a practice and tradition I was taught while I was in India studying Ayurveda.

Nasal Breathing Tips:

1. If your child snores, has chronic congestion, or simply cannot breathe through the nose for some reason, do not give up. Try kid's "breathe-right" strips available at any pharmacy or grocery store. They increase the opening of the nasal passages by 30% and can be a great help to a nasal breather-in-training.

2. If your child produces excessive mucus, you can try having him or her sniff a saline nasal spray to rinse out and clean the sinuses. After rinsing, take a cotton swab and dip it in vegetable oil (cold-pressed sesame oil or other high-quality vegetable oil), and swab the child's nasal passages with the oil. Your child should then sniff two or three times to draw the oil into the sinuses. The oil lubricates the dry and irritated sinuses and can make nasal breathing much easier to learn.

Back to the Future

While I was studying Ayurveda in India, I went hiking with a man who was somewhere between 75 and 80 years old. He was an expert in Ayurveda and yoga. We were hiking in the Himalayan foothills in search of some rare herbs. It was a hot day and a strenuous hike. On the steep trail, in spite of all my endurance training as a runner, I was huffing and puffing. But this very vital elderly man was gliding up the side of the mountain, breathing through his nose as if he were standing still. His breathing pattern was neither fast nor labored, but it was long, slow, and somewhat loud. It was a distinct sound, and it compelled me to notice his breathing style. Here at the top of the mountain I was first introduced to the extraordinary benefits of nasal breathing.

The use of nasal breathing to enhance endurance has been practiced for thousands of years by many cultures across the world. Many of the original martial arts brought to China from India by the Buddhist monk Bodhidarma utilized methods of nasal breathing. The Vedic literature from India includes volumes of text detailing the value and benefits of nasal breathing practices. Pre-Columbian

Native Americans used techniques similar to those found in Eastern martial arts to train the great runners who maintained the sophisticated network of "mail runners" extending from Central America through South America. In ancient times, training athletes how to breathe was as important as training their physical structure.

Young runners or martial artists were asked by their elders to run to the top of a mountain and back with a handful of pebbles in their mouth. If you ever try running with pebbles in your mouth, you will quickly realize that the only way you can breathe is through your nose. Other stories tell of young runners who were required to take a mouthful of water at the beginning of a long run and spit that same water out at the end as part of their nasal-breathing training. These extreme techniques were designed to force the body to breathe more efficiently, and as a result, be able to perform physical feats of endurance and strength that were beyond the limits we recognize today.

The Tarahumara of northern Mexico are one of the last remaining running tribes. Their name for themselves, *Raramuri,* or "light feet," is not just figurative. They regularly run an average of 50 to 75 miles a day and routinely complete runs of 150 miles with ease. When they enter road races like the Leadville 100, the highest altitude 100-mile race in the U.S., held in Leadville, Colorado, they amaze everyone with their ability. Western medical researchers have studied these runners and have concluded that what they witnessed was not humanly possible.

When the researchers asked the Tarahumara runners to complete a 26-mile marathon, the Tarahumara laughed at the distance, regarding it as child's play. In the scorching heat and rough mountainous terrain of the Chihuahua desert of northern Mexico, these runners ran the 26 miles at an average pace of 6 miles per hour. World-class marathoners run at an average pace of more than 10 miles per hour, so the Tarahumara's speed was not remarkable. The most amazing thing about their running physiology was when they finished the marathon, their heart rates averaged 130 beats per minute compared to the 160 to 180 beats per minute that most marathoners average. What was even more astounding was that their blood pressure was actually lower at the end of the run than it was before they started running.

The scientists were most surprised by the fact that their subjects' breathing was as calm and easy at the end of their run as if they had been standing still and not running at all. In addition to these amazing facts, the Tarahumara's best runners are in their 50s. It is natural for their running ability to improve with age, something we in the West cannot explain.

Today, only 11 years since the publication of *Body, Mind, and Sport,* compelling new research indicating that there *is* a difference between nasal breathing and mouth breathing. The difference is substantial, and the benefits of nasal breathing are so important that every parent must know how to teach their children to breathe through their nose.

Kids Breathe in the Strangest Ways

When my children were infants, I noticed that they seemed to breathe only through their noses. Their mouths were designated for eating and sucking—just about everything in sight—and their noses were exclusively for breathing. I noticed this quite dramatically when one of my small children caught a cold and developed sinus congestion, making it difficult for him to breathe through his nose. I watched him lie in bed snorting through his nose as he unsuccessfully attempted to fill his lungs. He was still breathing, although not very fully, so it was not a breathing emergency; but I remember wishing that I could teach him how to breathe through his mouth. I just wanted him to be able to open his mouth and fill his lungs.

After this experience, I called a pediatrician friend of mine and asked him about infant breathing mechanisms. He said that infants are considered to be obligate nasal breathers, which means that they lack the ability to breathe through their mouths. This was in the early 1990s, and since that time, medical science has redefined infants from being obligate nasal breathers to being preferred nasal breathers, meaning that the nose is the breathing apparatus of choice, but not the only choice.

If an infant's nose becomes completely obstructed, he or she will begin to suffocate. At this point, the body sounds the emergency alarm. The child starts to cry, gasping for air through the mouth. This crying is functional because it delivers large quantities of air into the lungs to deal with the emergency at hand. Crying also triggers the secretion of copious amounts of mucus in an attempt to drain the sinuses and restore normal nasal breathing. Once the sinuses are clear and nasal breathing can be resumed, the panic button is switched off and the crying stops.

Breathing while crying or breathing through the mouth shunts the air to the upper lobes of the lungs. This is where most of the lungs' stress receptors and the connections to the sympathetic nervous system—the "fight or flight" response—are located. Imagine for a moment what would happen if you came face-to-face with a bear in the woods. Your initial response would most likely be a gasping, fear-based mouth breath. This gasping breath fills the upper lobes of the lungs first, which activates the stress receptors and engages the fight or flight response. Ideally, this would happen quickly enough for you to get a burst of energy and speed to save your life.

It is not necessary to see a bear and gasp for air, nor to cry, to activate these stress receptors in the upper chest. The act of shallow breathing alone will activate a stress response, even when a major threat does not exist. Our approximately 26,000 daily breaths can have a profound effect. If all, or a majority, of those 26,000 breaths are shallow, upper-chest mouth breaths, then the stress receptors of the sympathetic nervous system will be the ones which are primarily activated. This constant activation of the emergency or stress response in the body triggers an excessive and unnecessary production of degenerative stress hormones.

Breathing through the nose, on the other hand, delivers the air deeper into the lower lobes of the lungs because of the structure inside the nasal passages and sinus cavities. The inside of the nose is not a simple tube or open cavern, but contains turbinates, which act like turbines. I remember when I saw a set of horse turbinates. Horses are large, obligate nasal breathers, which means they cannot breathe through their mouths. When I looked at the horse's skull, I was struck by the turbinates in the side of the head: they looked like big conch shells with spiraling passages essential to accelerate the air all the way to the lungs—quite a long distance in a horse. Human turbinates are smaller, yet still every bit as dramatic. These turbines allow the air to spin and move in a thin, rotating stream. This more forceful and direct stream of air effectively penetrates the deeper, lower lobes of the lungs.

Rock-a-Bye Baby:

A screaming, mouth-breathing child is instantly calmed when nursing. This is illustrated in *stillen,* the German word for breast-feeding, meaning to still or quiet the child. When babies nurse, they are forced to breathe through their noses. The turbinates allow the air to be directed deeper into the lungs, soothing the child by activating the parasympathetic nervous system.

Breathing into the lower lobes of the lungs is preferred because we find 60% to 80% of the lungs' blood supply waiting for oxygen delivery and gas exchange. The receptors for the parasympathetic nervous system are concentrated in the lower lobes of the lungs. Nasal breathing, because of its connection with the lower lobes of the lungs, activates the polar opposite response of the upper-chest mouth breathing.

Differences between the parasympathetic and sympathetic nervous system:

Parasympathetic	Sympathetic
Relaxation response in body	Fight or flight, activates body
Connected to lower lobes of lungs	Connected to upper lung lobes
Increased immunity/digestion	Inhibition of digestion/immunity
Rejuvenating	Depletes body
Decreases heart rate	Increases heart rate

Decreases blood sugar   Increases blood sugar
Nasal breathing   Mouth breathing

Lions and Tigers and Bears, Oh My!

As your children grow up, start school, and begin to endure the peer pressures, social tension, and stresses of childhood, their breathing tends to change dramatically. Instead of having the relaxed life of infants or toddlers—who naturally breathe deeply—their breathing becomes more constricted due to increasing stress. The daily pressures of life can be like coming upon a bear in the woods. With each experience of having to perform on the soccer field, in the classroom and hallways, and on the playground, children take fear-based gasping breaths into their chest. Children who have been taught to breathe deeply and efficiently through the nose have an advantage because they will have a better ability to handle stress than a shallow mouth-breathing schoolmate.

I remember one summer watching my children standing by a swimming pool and noticing that the size of their lower abdomens steadily decreased as they got older. As they aged, they sadly learned to "suck it up" and endure the woes of childhood. My 2-year-old had a body posture that revealed he was the king of the world with the biggest belly of the lot. He, out of all the kids, felt the most comfortable letting his belly just hang out. His lower ribs moved out to the side as he breathed, and all the movement in his body allowed him to breathe deeply, naturally, and efficiently into the lower lobes of the lungs. My 5-year-old, on the other hand, was on the front lines of social and school stress; he was daily meeting the bear in the woods. Clearly, my 5-year-old had started breathing more in the upper chest as both a survival mechanism and a response to the stress of childhood. Any parent will confirm that kids are not overly considerate of each other's feelings, so that getting their feelings hurt is the rule rather than the exception. My 7- and 9-year-olds held their stomachs even tighter as an indication of even more controlled breathing.

Why Does Sucking It In and Enduring Life Affect the Breath?

With each exhale, the ribs naturally squeeze the lungs through the muscular effort called elastic recoil in order to more fully and efficiently move air out. This process is extremely vulnerable to stress. Just as we gasp when we see a bear, if a child is under stress, the body responds by breathing shallowly into the upper chest only, where the stress receptors of the lungs are located. Meanwhile, the lower lobes of the lungs are being held even more tightly with each exhalation. The lower lobes succumb to the elastic recoil of the ribs, becoming tight and rigid.

This creates a positive feedback loop. More stress leads to more shallow breathing, and continuing to breathe shallowly leads to feelings of increased stress; the lower lobes become even more rigid and inaccessible. The elastic recoil mechanism of the ribs creates further rigidity in the lower rib cage and the lower lungs. Soon the rib cage literally becomes a cage squeezing the heart and lungs and forcing all the breath into the upper chest. Breathing only into the upper chest continues to stimulate the sympathetic nervous system or the stress response.

> Life for a child soon becomes an immune-compromising survival emergency.

Each of these upper-chest stress breaths tells the body to trigger a stress-fighting hormonal response from the adrenals—which will save your child's life when necessary, give your child the extra boost in a race or competition, or provide the extra focus to complete a test or a tough assignment—but on a regular basis, this stress brings with it a degenerative and disease-producing biochemistry. Stress hormones produce free radicals as waste products, which we now recognize to be the leading cause of aging, chronic disease, cancer, and even death. And, on a more immediate basis, the biochemistry of constant stress affects your child's moods and happiness. When your child begins to breathe more naturally, deeper into the lower lobes of the lungs, it activates the parasympathetic nervous system, the body's calming response, allowing the child to handle stress by letting it glide right over them like water off a duck's back. When your child is able to handle stress in this way, it does not impact or penetrate the nervous system or deplete the immune system.

The Rib Cage or the Rib Massage

The ribs are actually designed to be twelve pairs of levers that move in a coordinated manner to massage the heart and the lungs with each breath. This massage supports lymphatic circulation. The movement also massages the muscles along the spine and shoulders and the associated organs of the chest, the heart and lungs, with each of the 26,000 breaths your child takes each day. When the lower rib cage becomes stiff and rigid, full breathing becomes more difficult and deep breathing will not take place until the lower rib cage again becomes resilient and accessible to nasal breathing.

Our bodies' natural response to stress and the impact of the elastic recoil of the rib cage makes maintaining the flexibility of the rib cage and free and clear access to the lower lobes of the lungs difficult. This is why ancient runners would train with pebbles or water in their mouths to force them to be aware of their nasal breathing. As parents, we have a great opportunity to teach our children to breathe deeply and efficiently through the stressful years of childhood. Regaining nasal breathing access to the lower lobes of the lungs is not difficult; it just takes a little practice. I have been teaching athletes and non-athletes alike to breathe this way for almost 20 years and I have seen miracles.

> Deep nasal breathing facilitates a feeling of calm that I call the eye of the storm. In the eye of the storm, the child is trained to handle skillfully many diverse and stressful situations on the outside while on the inside maintaining internal peace and calm.

On the battlefield in the epic poem, *The Mahabharata*, Krishna revealed the secret of victory to the great warrior, Arjuna. He said, *"Yogastha kuru karmani,"* which means, first establish yourself in being, then perform action. The point he was making is that one must first capture the experience of inner calm or *being,* and only then can a person prevail in the action of victory. It is like the hurricane effect—the bigger the eye or the calm of the storm, the more powerful the winds. Billie Jean King summed it up perfectly as she described a competitive arena as, "a perfect combination of violent action taking place in an atmosphere of *total* tranquility."

 Secret 10: The tenth secret to health is to practice nasal breathing. Nasal breathing yields not only health and performance benefits, it is a key ingredient in the development and full use of the nervous system and the ability to access the subtle and spiritual energy of the body.

David and Goliath

Let's discuss the impact nasal breathing can have on a child's enjoyment of exercise and life.

In the 1990s I trained the coaches of a small private high school in the Midwest in the methods of using nasal-breathing techniques during their sports training. The soccer team at that time was small, inexperienced, and one of the weakest teams in the league. Actually, I don't think they won a game in the entire season—or did they? Is winning determined only by the final score? Something happened to the team when they started practicing nasal-breathing techniques. Their focus quite naturally moved from winning the game to enjoying the game. The goal orientation that is usually an integral part of high school competitive sports was replaced with a process orientation, or a focus on playing the game itself. This change in focus allowed the team to improve their ability and skill level without stressing over achievement.

Their new approach and attitude made a big difference in the team's experience of the game they played against the most dominant and powerful team in the league. In this competition, the stronger team beat them handily, winning by 8–0, but the inexperienced team had expected a 20-goal defeat.

During this "slaughter," the young and inexperienced players found a way to enjoy the process of the match. From their

> Winning does not always mean scoring more goals, and the winner is not always the one who scores more points. In this case, the win was celebrated in the hearts of the team who may have scored fewer goals—but clearly won the battle.

perspective, they were actually playing quite well and were proud of their performance. As the game went on, the players enjoyed themselves, even in defeat. They showed great sportsmanship and an overwhelming enthusiasm while playing. The joy of the battle and the enthusiasm the losing team showed actually frustrated the more dominant team to the point that it affected their ability to play.

At the game's end, the losing team celebrated their defeat as if it were a huge victory. This infuriated the winning team. For some reason, the winning team gleaned no satisfaction from their triumph. They became so irritated by the response of the losing team that they actually challenged them to a rematch. They figured that if they played them again they could not only score more points but also destroy the other team's morale.

When the "losing" team heard the challenge of a rematch, they just laughed and celebrated even more.

How is it that breathing through the nose could create this type of psychology on the soccer field? To answer this question, in 1992, we studied the effects of nasal breathing during exercise. Ten high school students breathed through their nose during a submaximal exercise-bike ergometer stress test. We then had the same students do the same task while breathing through their mouth and compared the results. We measured heart rates, breath rates, level of perceived exertion, brain waves, blood pressure, and the impact on the sympathetic and parasympathetic nervous systems.

As the body endured higher levels of vigorous exercise, the nasal-breathing exercisers handled the stress with significantly more ease than the mouth breathers. One of the indications for this was the rate of breath while exercising. The nasal breathers rode the exercise bike at the high level of resistance—200 watts—with a breath rate of only 14 breaths per minute. This is significant when you realize that the average breath rate at rest is 16 to 18 breaths per minute. Imagine exercising on at a vigorous pace while breathing four breaths per minute slower than you do at rest.

During the mouth-breathing test the next day, the same group of kids exercising at the same level of exertion were huffing and puffing at an amazing 48 breaths per minute. This is a huge difference: mouth breathers had a rate of 48 breaths per minute while nasal breathers performed the same exercise with only 14 breaths per minute (see Graph A).

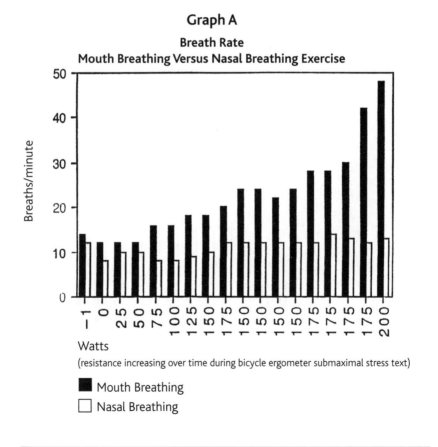

Graph A: Mouth Breathing Versus Nasal Breathing During Exercise

When we asked the participants how they felt while exercising and mouth breathing as compared to exercising and nasal breathing, the results were even more impressive. To answer this question, the high

> In other words, they were able to transform their subjective response to intense and vigorous exercise by 60%!

school students were asked to use a Borg scale of perceived exertion to rate their comfort levels on a scale of one to ten with ten being the highest and most exhaustive level of exertion (see Graph B). When they were mouth breathing with the resistance at the highest level, they all reported an exertion and exhaustion level of ten. But the perceived exertion level changed dramatically when the

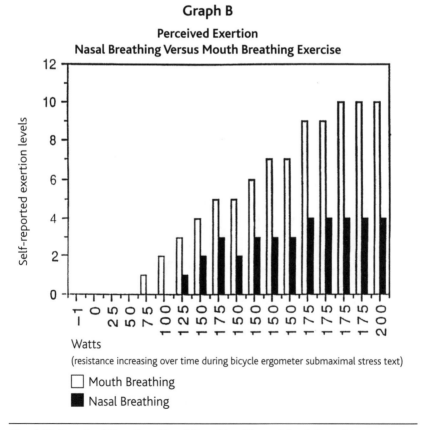

Graph B

Perceived Exertion
Nasal Breathing Versus Mouth Breathing Exercise

Watts

(resistance increasing over time during bicycle ergometer submaximal stress text)

☐ Mouth Breathing
■ Nasal Breathing

Graph B: Perceived Exertion: Nasal Breathing Versus Mouth Breathing same students were nasal breathing and performed the same exercise at the same high level of resistance. In this case, their perceived exertion level was only four instead of the previous level of ten.

> Imagine accomplishing the same amount of work and handling the same amount of stress in your life, but instead of feeling maxed-out at a perceived exertion level of ten, you are handling your work effortlessly with a perceived exertion level of four? This is analogous to how the nasal breathing students felt in the exercise study.

When I ask people in my seminars how they feel they are handling the stress in their lives on a scale of one to ten, the majority tell me that they are living life at a constant ten. If nasal breathing changed the perceived exertion for the students in the exercise study, it just might change how we view our levels of perceived exertion—stress and distress—in our daily lives.

Most of the stress-combatting techniques we learn as adults reduce stress *after* it has already occurred and has had a debilitating impact on our bodies and minds. By using breathing techniques and making them a way of life, we can teach children how to *prevent* the impacts of stress. If we show our children now how to remain calm in stressful situations, they will be able to gracefully and effortlessly handle levels of even more extreme stress as adults without being subject to its the immune-compromising, disease-producing and mood-destabilizing physiological effects.

We need to teach our children how to deal with stress and cope with fearful conditions. It is a part of growing up in modern times. But it is also important to remember that even though mouth breathing may be associated with a fear-based state, that does not mean it is always bad. In fact, mouth breathing is as natural a way of breathing as

If we can teach our children to handle the stress of daily life with this level of peace and calm, we will be doing them a service and sending them off into the world with a skill that is more valuable than learning to how to drive or swim.

nasal breathing. But if children grow up breathing predominantly through their mouth, they may lose the ability to breathe through their nose, sentencing them to 26,000 stress-inducing breaths each day whether or not they are under any stress. In this chapter, my goal is to educate parents about the benefits of nasal breathing while sleeping and exercising.

Breathing Brain Waves

To further examine the effects of nasal breathing on the body, we measured brain-wave function during both the nasal- and mouth-breathing exercises. There are four different frequencies, or states, of brain waves that correspond to different types of mental activities. These are Beta, Alpha Theta, and Delta waves. Beta brain waves are associated with the active, working, thinking mind and typically prevail when the body is under stress. Alpha brain waves are typically seen during states of relaxation, calm, focus, and in meditation or while practicing mind-body disciplines like yoga. Theta waves are associated with the subconscious mind. THey are present in dreaming sleep and deep meditative states and are a source of creative and spiritual connection. Finally, Delta waves are the slowest and most relaxed, are seen during deep sleep and hypnosis. Delta waves are associated with the unconscious mind, intuition, empathy, and with an accepting and absorbing mental disposition.

When we exercise, adrenaline and other stress hormones are released to allow the body to perform strenuous activity, and the corresponding brain waves (predominantly Beta) often become fast and incoherent. During the mouth-breathing exercise study, this is exactly what we saw (see Graph C). But the brain waves of the people who were nasal breathing during exercise showed calm and coherent patterns. This means the brain as a whole was communicating and functioning in a coordinated fashion. Rather than the brain waves becoming faster with increased Beta activity as expected, the brain actually slowed down and bursts of Alpha waves were measured (see Graph D). Alpha waves are rarely seen during aerobic exercise, but have been seen in mind-body exercise and in yoga, which have a very different effect on the body.

Graph C: Predominant Beta-Wave Activity
Brain-Wave Activity During Mouth Breathing Exercise

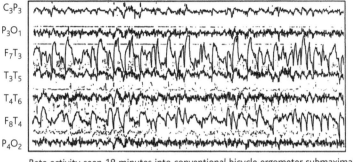

Beta activity seen 18 minutes into conventional bicycle ergometer submaximal stress test (comparable in time to 11 minutes of "Listening Phase")

*large waves in F7T3, F8T4 are due to eye movements

Graph C: Brain-Wave Activity During Mouth Breathing Exercise

Graph D: Predominant Alpha-Wave Activity
Brain-Wave Activity During Nasal Breathing Exercise

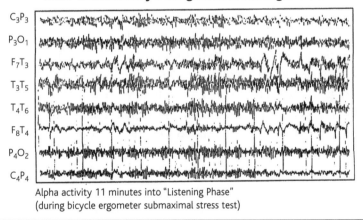

Alpha activity 11 minutes into "Listening Phase"
(during bicycle ergometer submaximal stress test)

Graph D: Brain-Wave Activity During Nasal Breathing Exercise

During vigorous exercise, we were able to trigger a state of relaxation and calm euphoria through the use of the breath. The same brain-wave activity you see during meditation and deep relaxation is what we reproduced with these students who were completing a physically demanding aerobic exercise but breathing through their nose. This state of relaxation, as indicated by the predominance of

> Instead of responding to exercise as a life-threatening, stressful emergency, nasal breathing facilitates an experience that is calm, enjoyable, and stress-free.

Alpha waves measured, explains why the children perceived the exertion to be at a level of four during the nasal-breathing exercise as compared to ten during mouth-breathing exercise.

Children are born to breathe naturally through their noses unless subjected to stress and a constant "bear in the woods" state of mind. When children are retrained in how to breathe through the nose during exercise (which is typically perceived by the body as a stressful experience), the state of their mind during the exercise is dramatically transformed.

We searched through the previous 20 years of brain-wave research and could not find any other studies that showed the production of Alpha brain-wave activity during aerobic exercise.

Catch That Brain Wave

Recent studies investigating the changes in brain-wave activity throughout child development paint an interesting picture for trying to understand what makes your child tick. Research by Laibow in 1999 showed that in the first 5 years of life, your child's brain-wave activity is dominated by Delta and Theta waves. Remember that the slow Delta waves are associated with sleep, hypnosis, and the unconscious, and since they are related to an attitude of acceptance and mental absorption, they are connected to the time in a child's life when he or she is new to the world and taking everything in.

Between the ages of 2 and 6, slightly faster Theta waves predominate. These waves often signal the state of consciousness found between waking and sleeping. I'm sure most parents have witnessed this state in their children when they are half asleep.

Around age 6, brain waves speed up slightly and express Alpha states of consciousness, represented by the calm we saw during the nasal-breathing exercise study. If we are lucky, our children will fall into the natural equanimity represented by Alpha states.

Beta waves—which are associated with the thinking mind, focus and concentration, and increased levels of activity and stress—do not make a full appearance until age 10 or 12.

Throughout their development children make a mental journey, as well as a physical one. As infants and young children, they start out with a mind that is predominantly slow, non-thinking, impressionable, and accepting. During these first few years of life, children are experiencing the Delta and Theta states. Then they move into Alpha states, in which they still possess the childlike brain activity of play, relaxation, and calm. Children do not lose the brain waves of innocence and play until they move into expressing Beta-wave activity around the age of 10 or 12. It is only then that they have the more analytical functioning optimal for academic study.

> Adults can and do produce all of these brain-wave frequencies during activities associated with the particular states. Adults who exhibit predominantly Beta waves are able to calm the mind and produce slower, more coherent, and more highly sophisticated brain waves through the practice of meditation, biofeedback, relaxation techniques, yoga, and other mind-body disciplines. Both children and adults can use techniques like nasal breathing and participation in mind-body and relaxation-based activities to facilitate calmer and more peaceful states of mind.

We have amazing opportunities with children to develop and facilitate these brain waves and associated brain functions. Our study showed that a coherent pattern of Alpha brain-wave activity can be produced during a stressful session of vigorous exercise in 16-year-olds, at a developmental time when their brains are functioning in a state of primarily Beta-wave activity. Imagine a child who is able to pass through the stresses of childhood in an environment conducive to and supporting the slower and more highly sophisticated Alpha-, Theta-, and Delta-brain wave activity.

This explains why, in the story I related earlier, members of the weaker soccer team gained such pleasure from a process-oriented experience even though they did not score as many points. When the mind and body are coordinated through the use of nasal breathing and the subsequent production of Alpha waves, the experience is clearly less stressful, and the feelings of struggle and work come to be replaced by playfulness and joy. Children can once again enjoy physical activity for its own sake and not have to be pushed or motivated to exercise by outside forces.

> If children are left alone, they will play tirelessly for hours in the same way tiger or bear cubs play. Kids never call it exercise or a workout: they are hard at play. Try to keep up with a bunch of 7- and 8-year-olds at play and not only will you will get the best workout of your life—you may learn a thing or two about having fun.

The Power of Play

Many great people speak about the power of play. Baseball Hall-of-Famer Willie Stargell of the Pittsburg Pirates said:

> "The secret to my success is that I don't go out to work, I go out to play."

The Kenyan running team trained with an unwritten philosophy:

> "Run everyday from youth on and run so you will enjoy it the next day. Everything else will follow automatically."

This kind of play, which is so desperately lacking in our culture, is an essential ingredient for child development. During these states of play, there exists not only an increased enjoyment of the activity but an optimal learning opportunity for children.

In the book *Magical Parent, Magical Child,* by Michael Mendizza and Joseph Chilton Pearce, Pearce says:

> "Some parents think it is a jungle out there. We need to raise a tough child to succeed and survive in that jungle world. New brain research shows why this notion has not worked well for anyone, child, adult or society. The best survival in a jungle is to be intelligent, balanced, self-reliant, resourceful and happy. Then one finds not a jungle but a playground wherever one is.

Play is the child's royal road to intelligence, creative thinking, and joy. The child who can play will play skillfully and successfully throughout life. People complain that all children to want to do is play. Nature designs children that way. And nature intends, as children mature into adults, to retain their childlike qualities of wonder and lifelong joy of learning. When a child grows and becomes the parent, it is precisely these childlike qualities that will transform parenting into one of life's most powerful learning experiences imaginable."

Mendizza says:

"The state athletes call the zone, what the researchers and professionals refer to as the flow and what children call play share selfless absorption and complete engagement in the moment. We believe this state of complete unconflicted behavior is nature's baseline, her expectation, for optimal learning, performance, and well-being."

It's Playtime!

Most of all children need ample time just to play. This time is not your children's piano lessons, soccer practice, or gymnastics; it is time every day when your children can enjoy free and unstructured play. It is in this fun environment of recreational play that your children will learn, develop, grow, and mature more rapidly than they will by engaging in any other activity. Play triggers an optimal leaning experience for children as well as mood-stabilizing endorphins that will balance their biochemistry. Their memories of the freedom of play will linger throughout their lives as a reminder that there is a little kid alive and well within them.

When I talk about play I mean running around outside playing games—preferably play that brings them joy. Our children are overloaded with TV and video games that have created an artificial need for stimulation that is hard to satisfy with "hide and seek." Blowing up buildings and leaping across chasms on a video screen is an addictive stimulation that is a hard act to follow with backyard play.

> Remember the old saying: a child who plays well can never grow dull!

What indoor, stationary games do not provide is the biochemical, full-body activation of endorphins; the improvement of the circulatory system, which brings better health and increased oxygenation of the muscles, organs, and other tissues; movement of toxins out of the deep tissues of the body for elimination; socialization; and the integration of body and mind, which helps children develop to their full potential. For children, running around and participating in active games develops coordination and self-confidence and helps to prevent the epidemic of obesity that is rampant in the United States. Countless studies show that physical activity can help reduce the risk of degenerative diseases like type-II diabetes and cardiovascular disease. Active play also stimulates the immune system, keeping children running down the road of perfect health.

Play and the Lymphatic System

Play and exercise are crucial for the healthy functioning of the lymphatic and immune systems. I have talked a great deal so far about other aspects of the lymphatic system and the importance of hydration, massage, and proper elimination. What I have not yet touched on is the mechanism by which the lymphatic fluid moves through the vessels. Our heart actively pumps blood through the body. But the lymphatic system does not have its own pump, and the heart does not serve as its pump. Some of the larger lymphatic vessels are muscular and can contract on their own to push the lymphatic fluid along, but the majority of the lymphatic vessels rely on our muscles to move fluid through them.

The vessels and tubes of the lymphatic system are found predominantly tucked within our active, voluntary skeletal muscles. When these muscles contract while we walk, move, or exercise, they squeeze the lymphatic vessels, pumping fluids through the system, effectively removing toxins and waste products, and ensuring that the immune system has circulatory access to every cell in the body.

The Health Benefits of Nasal Breathing

There health benefits of nasal breathing as compared to mouth breathing pay dividends both during the day and while resting. The nasal passages and mucous membranes will warm and moisturize the air headed for the lungs via the bronchioles. If the air is properly warmed and moisturized, the bronchioles will maintain a proper balance (not too much mucus and not too little) and immunity remains intact.

When air is taken in only through the mouth, it is neither warmed nor moisturized. The air tends to dry the mucous membranes and shocks and irritates the respiratory tract and bronchioles. Air that moves through the nasal passages is also filtered, so if there are any pollens, pollutants, or chemical irritants in the air, mouth breathing can exacerbate the situation. The mucous membranes will react by producing excess mucus, which can get trapped or remain stagnant in the sinuses or bronchioles and act as a perfect breeding ground for a bacterial or viral infection.

The mouth is a quick emergency route for the breath, which triggers a crisis mode neurology and biochemistry that compromise immunity and are degenerative for the body. The mouth does not contain a filter, so the air is not moisturized, warmed, or prepared in any way to access the deeper lobes of the lungs. As a result the mouth-breathing air stream is much thicker and simply cannot penetrate the lower, more delicate lobes of the lungs. Because the nose is a longer breathing apparatus, it is the body's first choice for breathing when stress is absent.

A Denver study measured the fatigue associated with the common cold. The researchers discovered that the reason people felt fatigued when they had a cold was that blocked sinuses made it impossible to breathe through the nose. Lack of nasal breathing created an oxygen deficit that resulted in tiredness and fatigue.

Miracle Molecule

In 1998, the Nobel Prize in Physiology and Medicine was awarded jointly to Robert Furchgott, Louis Ignarro, and Fred Nurad for their groundbreaking research on how the nitric oxide molecule acts as a messenger in the human body. Nitric oxide is a toxic gas that comes from car exhausts, acid rain, and air pollution and is responsible for destroying the ozone layer. In large quantities this gas is poisonous to humans and toxic to the environment, but in very small quantities it is nothing short of a panacea. According to the trio's research, minute amounts of nitric oxide are produced in the body and are responsible for physiological processes that provide a host of health benefits. The research was so impressive, that in 1992 nitric oxide was named the "Molecule of the Year" by *Science,* which called it the hottest and most exciting thing in neurobiology.

Nitric oxide is a gas that in the body acts as a neurotransmitter, an immunoregulator, and a vasodilator. It is responsible for a host of functions that promote health, such as:

- Regulating blood pressure,
- Stimulating and activating the immune system,
- Killing cancer cells and microorganisms like bacteria and viruses,
- Increasing blood supply to cells through dilation of arteries and bronchioles,
- Aiding in muscular control, balance and coordination,
- Contributing to the mechanisms involved in long-term memory.

Nitric oxide was shown to protect the body against:

- Cardiovascular disease
- Parkinson's disease
- Alzheimer's disease
- Diabetic neuropathy
- Impotence

Since nitric oxide was identified as a signaling molecule in 1989, there have been thousands of studies extolling its remarkable physiological effects. In a study published in the *Japanese Journal of Physiology,* nitric oxide production during exercise was compared while nasal breathing and mouth breathing. The study found that breathing through the nasal passages caused the production of a significantly higher amount of nitric oxide than was produced during mouth breathing. As the exercise intensity increased with nasal breathing, so did nitric oxide levels. This study indicated that during nasal-breathing exercise the excess nitric oxide produced delivered a host of health benefits that did not occur during exercise while breathing through the mouth.

The same study also found that at least 50% of the nitric oxide found in exhaled air was produced in the nasal passages. Another study, by the American Physiological Society, found that nitric oxide is not only produced, but it is also absorbed, in the nose, indicating that during nasal-breathing exercise, the health benefits of nitric oxide production and absorption are maximized. A study done in Sweden at the Karolinska Hospital confirms these results: levels of nitric oxide are higher in the nose than in the mouth, especially during inhalation. This concentration of nitric oxide increases the levels of oxygenation in the lungs and bloodstream.

Ten years ago, any talk of linking nasal breathing with science was dismissed as quackery. The scientific acceptance of new ideas has come a long way since then. What is interesting is that these are not new ideas at all; they are, in fact, over 5,000 years old and have been practiced continuously throughout the centuries.

So … How To Breathe Through the Nose While Exercising

It seems like we start panting and puffing almost the moment we or our children start running or exercising. Breathing through the nose while physically exerting oneself aerobically may appear at first to be an impossible task. The trick is to build up slowly, just as you build up endurance in any other way. This means that if your children are already very active and used to running or playing sports, they may have to slow way down from their usual pace in order to be able to nasal breathe. Remember, it is important not to force this, or any other practice, on your children.

> My 15-year-old daughter now finishes all of her endurance runs in first place. She tells me that if she opens her mouth she gets out of breath and can't run.

I often suggest to people that they begin their nasal breathing practice while walking. You can also train your children to nasal breathe by going for walks together, continuing the 5,000-year-old Ayurvedic tradition of teaching nasal breathing by example. I have been casually telling my kids to nasal breathe since they were very young, and I have watched them pick up on nasal breathing by going for runs with me. Like the Tarahumara, who break the monotony of running by kicking a little ball, I usually take a tennis ball and a kid or two and go for a nasal-breathing, "mini-soccer-ball" run. As we pass the ball back and forth, we play the game of keeping the ball with us and breathing through our noses. My kids have learned by imitating me—not by me formally teaching or training them. It works!

Start out at a walking pace that you and your child can comfortably maintain while continuing to breathe through the nose. Slowly, over time, start to increase the pace, but only to the point where nasal breathing can still be maintained. If the pace becomes too rapid, slow down until the nasal breathing catches up again. As the body's stamina increases over time, and as the lungs and the nervous system get used to this new way of breathing, you can start to practice nasal breathing while hiking, running, and participating in other activities. Over time, your child will soon develop a preference for nasal breathing.

As your children get older they may want to read my book, *Body, Mind, and Sport,* which offers nasal-breathing training techniques for all sports and types of exercise.

> Our job as parents is to lead our children to "water." Kids know what is right for them, and when they are "thirsty" they will drink. Sometimes you might not think they have drunk the water, and then months or years later you will find that when you weren't looking, they drank it all!

Nasal Breathing and the Mind

Both modern medicine and the 5,000-year-old sciences of Ayurveda and yoga describe the nasal-breathing cycle. Throughout the day and night, the dominance of the flow of the breath naturally alternates between the nostrils, changing approximately every one and a half to three hours. According to the descriptions of the subtle physiology of the body in Ayurveda and yoga, two of the body's primary *nadis*, or subtle channels of the nervous system, flow through the nostrils and connect the nose to the brain. The *nadi* flowing through the right nostril connects to the left hemisphere of the brain and the *nadi* flowing through the left nostril connects to the right hemisphere. So, not only are the nose and brain connected on a very physical level through smell and the olfactory nerve, they are connected on a subtle level as well, through the *nadis*.

The description of this connection is not limited to Ayurveda. Recent medical and physiological research suggests that there is not only a demonstrable cycle in the physical act of air moving through the nostrils, but also a cycle of alternating cerebral dominance between the hemispheres in the brain. This cycle has been demonstrated in both humans and other mammals while waking and in sleep, as reported in the *International Journal of Neuroscience,* and cognitive ability in one hemisphere of the brain coordinates with forcing the breath through the nostril on the opposite side of the head. Researchers at Montana State University have also reported differences in cognitive performance related to the flow of air through specific nostrils, and studies done at the University of Toronto describe the effects on emotions of breathing through different nostrils. So breathing through the nose provides something else that breathing through the mouth cannot—a connection with the cerebral hemispheres of the frontal lobes: the cognitive, thinking part of our brain.

This is particularly significant in light of new research on mental health and the hemispheres of the frontal lobes. There is research that shows that in conditions such as depression or anxiety, one cerebral hemisphere of the brain is more active than the other. In many cases, the right hemisphere of the frontal lobe shows greater activation in anxiety, while the left hemisphere is more active in cases of depression. This has been measured in children, including studies done in 2002 by the Central Institute of Mental Health in Germany, which not only found differences in children with anxiety as compared to children without anxiety, but also differences in boys versus girls, and in children of different ages. Another study done at the same institute found patterns of asymmetry in children with ADHD. This is a very new area of study, but the healing power of nasal breathing may prove to be significant in these conditions.

The Ancient Science of Breath

Breath has been associated with life force throughout history and in cultures worldwide. In China, this life energy is called *chi;* in Japan it is called *ki;* and India it is called *prana*. Interestingly, the Greek word for breath is *pneuma,* which also means soul or spirit. In the martial arts, Zen archery, t'ai chi, chi gung, and yoga, the knowledge and control of one's *prana* is considered to be the key to mental and physical success. According to parameters of Western science, prana has yet to be measured. This is not to say prana does not exist, but that we have not yet developed an instrument subtle enough to measure it.

Prana, the body's life force, is carried into the body and to the cells through water, food, and air. This is why copious amounts of pure water, fresh well-cooked food, exercise, and breathing techniques are the fundamental components for perfect health.

Prana is carried by oxygen and enters the nasal cavity when you breathe. While in the nose, the air is cleaned, warmed, and filtered before it enters the sinuses and the lungs. It is said in Ayurveda that while the air is moving through the nose, prana moves through the olfactory plate directly into the emotional cortex or limbic system of the brain.

> Prana is the life force that exists in all living things such as plants, animals, our food and ourselves. Even the water that we drink can be devoid of or rich in prana.

Nasal breathing techniques are said to move prana and subtle energy into the brain and central nervous system.

During mouth breathing, the air and its associated prana are moved in and out of the body without entering the sinus cavity, resulting in less prana being absorbed into the brain and nervous system.

If exercise has the purpose of enhancing mind-body coordination, doesn't it make sense to access the brain and central nervous system first—and then access the rest of the body? With proper nasal breathing, not only is the amount of prana available to the nervous system increased, but it also directly accesses the brain. According to Ayurveda, the prana that enters the body through nasal breathing enters the control centers in the brain from which access to our full or enhanced human potential is initiated.

In the book, *Science Studies Yoga,* Dr. James Funderburks describes a 106-pound, 67-year-old yogi who exhibited incredible strength resulting from his yoga and breathing practices. The yogi strapped a 3/8-inch metal chain around his waist and feet. The chain was previously tested to be able to withstand 650 pounds of pressure without failing. After a few short nasal breaths, he exhaled and pushed his feet against the chain. It shattered.

The human body has unlimited potential. Einstein famously said that he used less than 10% of what he believed to be his full mental capacity. Some modern researchers now think that we only use .01% of our potential brainpower. The hardware we were born with is truly amazing: conservative estimates indicate that there are over 100 trillion neuronal junctions, or synapses, in the human brain. The speeds of transmission of signals across these neuronal connections are measured in thousandths and ten-thousandths of a second. There is new evidence that suggests that each one of our thoughts affects all of our cells instantaneously. The tools for the maximum integration of our mind and body seem to be hardwired into the human body and brain.

We have so much natural ability, and it makes sense that we are supposed to use it to achieve our highest potential as humans. When we look at traditional peoples, it seems that their cultures have held onto knowledge and techniques that once gave access to full human potential. The Tarahumara run amazing distances. The original martial techniques were used to develop the body's full potential, and only monks with severe and strict spiritual disciplines were allowed access to them. Native American runners covered extremely long distances with pebbles or water in their mouths to train the body to breathe through the nose. This access takes focus and discipline, but it is worth the work and effort. In our modern culture of convenience, so much comes easily that we rarely are motivated to strive for greatness.

We can experience greatness vicariously by watching TV. But according to Ayurveda, vicarious greatness is not enough, because we have so much potential to develop. Toward this end, I have shared the ancient secret of breathing, whose benefits are just beginning to be understood by Western science.

Bible: Genesis 2:7

And the LORD God formed man of the dust of the ground, and breathed into his nostrils the breath of life; and man became a living soul.

Chapter 12

Perfect Mental Health

> Sticks and stones may break my
> bones but names will never hurt me.

I don't think anyone ever believes this child's adage is true. Kids are very aware that name-calling does hurt—in fact, a lot more than a stick or stone. Physical pain tends to heal quickly, and kids bounce back and are playing the next day as if nothing happened. When children's feelings are hurt, it can affect their development, behavior, and personality. Traumatic or repetitive hurt can change the course of their lives.

For children, hurt feelings or stress can come in many varieties. But whether it's intense emotional, mental, peer-based stress, sports-performance pressure, or family and sibling conflict, these stressors all have the same basic degenerative biochemistry. We now know that stress causes 80% of all disease; and although children may not necessarily come down with something just because of stress (the disease-causing effects of stress are cumulative throughout life), the impact of stress on their lives is often far greater than it is for adults.

When we are under stress, the adrenals produce increased levels of stress-fighting hormones like cortisol and adrenaline, which can save our lives in a crisis and improve our short-term performance to respond to emergencies. In order to pump us up for action, these hormones raise blood pressure, increase blood sugar, suppress the immune system, and inhibit digestion, all of which have a degenerative effect on the body if maintained on a long-term basis.

Stress hormones are needed for short bursts of activity and short-term problem solving. They were never meant to be produced 24/7.

We develop habits and learn coping skills to handle uncomfortable and stressful situations when we are children. Today, the brains of most Americans are hitting the hormonal "panic button" way too often. Many of us perceive daily life as a series of emergencies or as a struggle, and kids are "copycats." If they see Mom and Dad operating constantly on overload, they will do the same. When the emotional alarm goes off, the brain sends out an "all-points bulletin" to deliver all available sugar—or emergency fuel—to the brain. Cravings result, blood sugar levels rise and subsequently plummet, moods become unstable, and any available fat is stored under the mattress and locked away in the fat cells until someone tells the body the crisis has passed. Unfortunately, the all-clear message rarely gets sent, and as a result, we have become the fattest country in the world with the highest rates of chronic disease.

Childhood stress may have an even greater impact on children's emotional and social development. In the first 18 months of life, learning, socialization, and self-worth are extremely vulnerable to stress. Rejection is probably the major stress children experience. Children are constantly being judged in sports or P.E. class, by their test grades, and by their peers. Children naturally seek love; to obtain love they seek approval. When they feel accepted, they feel secure, and in a secure environment they can grow and develop physically, mentally, and emotionally.

Are we creating the optimal learning and developmental environment for our children? To help parents create the most optimal environment possible, I will share some time-tested ideas about child development from the Ayurvedic tradition.

The messages we send to our children as we interact with them throughout the day are powerful. Parents and teachers say "No" 18 times for every "Yes" when interacting with their children and students. Caregivers dish out a "No" every nine minutes. They constantly hear that they are doing something wrong. This perpetual disapproval and censure increases their insecurity and makes the demonstration of approval and love an exception to the rule.

Dirty Dish Towels

Poor communication skills are an insidious form of stress that directly compromises the health of your children and has a severe impact on their emotional well-being. To reduce this stress, children need to be taught how to *communicate with* their peers and siblings rather than *react* to them. Hurt feelings can breed anger and resentment, which quickly insinuate themselves into a large portion of children's conversations, particularly with their close friends and family. With six kids in our home, communication problems can easily escalate, making the lack of these essential skills intolerable.

Teaching my children how to communicate with feeling may be one of the most important things I have learned to do as a parent. I use a simple but powerful technique that re-educates children and adults in communicating directly, heart-to-heart, with the ones we love—and that can be just about everybody!

 This exercise helped my kids realize that how they feel—and how they express those feelings—can instantly spread either joy or anger throughout the house.

The First Time I Used the
Dirty Dish Towel Technique

One day, while I was downstairs in the kitchen I suddenly heard the sounds of fighting upstairs. I called up to my 5-year-old, "Mason!"

He barked back at me, "What!" with a tone of voice that said clearly: don't bother me right now, I am mad at everyone.

I immediately called everyone downstairs: the 12-, 10-, 8-, and 5-year-olds.

I reached into the dish towel drawer and took out ten dish towels. I handed out the dish towels so that each child was connected to me by a towel and so that each of them was connected to each other with a towel.

At this point they all looked at me as if I were a little crazy, so I explained what I had set out to do.

"The dish towels we are holding represent our relationships to one another. Each of us actually has two relationships; the first is the love we have for each other and the second, represented by the dish towels, shows how we relate to or communicate with each other. As for the love, yes, of course, it is not always expressed, and right now that relationship is probably clouded with your fighting and anger," I told them. I continued by saying, "Deep inside of us is the love that we have for each other, and that love is permanent. No matter what any of you do, I could never stop loving you.

"I know that you may not agree with what I am saying right now, but every one of you has that same love for each other, and that cannot change.

"There is a problem, though. The way you treat each other when you feel angry, hurt, resentful, and frustrated can dirty the towel—the relationship—you have with each other. If you let your dish towels get dirty and don't clean them, you could spend your entire life never experiencing the love that exists in this family."

I then turned to my 5-year old, Mason, and asked him, "How did you feel when your older brother Austin took away your toy?"

"I felt mad," Mason quickly replied.

"Before you felt mad, right after he took the toy away, how did you feel?" I asked again.

"I was sad."

"Mason, did you tell Austin that he hurt your feelings?"

"No," Mason answered. "I just got mad and punched him."

Next I asked Austin, "How did you feel when you got punched?"

Austin replied, "I felt hurt, and then I got even more mad and hit Mason back."

I went on, "Okay, soon you two were hitting each other. Then I called up to Mason, and he yelled at *me,* and then *my* feelings were hurt. So now, what if your sister Janaki [my 12-year-old daughter] came to me and asked me for money to go to a movie, what would I say?"

Their answer was unanimous, "You wouldn't give it to her."

I said, "I might even be mean to her for no reason, just like Mason was mean to me for no reason."

I turned their attention to the dish towels. "Now look at the towels you are holding. Austin put dirt on the dish towel between himself and Mason when he took away Mason's toy. Mason's feelings got hurt, and instead of communicating his feelings to Austin, he just put more dirt on the dish towel, more dirt into the relationship between himself and Austin. More dirt means less communication. Soon your communication totally broke down and you started fighting.

"When I called to Mason, who was the one I could hear yelling the loudest, he yelled at me. That put dirt on the dish towel between Mason and me. That dish towel represents the relationship between Mason and me."

I said, "Now I have hurt feelings because of that dirt. I am no different that you are. I can get hurt feelings too!

"What happens after I get hurt?" I asked them.

"You get mad," they told me.

I continued talking them through the point I was trying to make. "So when Janaki asked me for money for the movie, and I got mad at her, I put dirt on that towel, I put dirt on my relationship with her. Now I have dirt on my dish towel with Mason, *and* I have dirt on my dish towel with Janaki, *and* I still have hurt feelings.

"So with these hurt feelings I have, what if Mommy came up to me now and asked me to take out the garbage, how what I react?"

They all said, "You would get mad at her."

"And for no good reason," I added. "What should I have done when Mason yelled at me?"

They said, "You should have told Mason how he made you feel."

"That's right," I said. "Now Austin," I asked, "if Mason would have told you how much you hurt his feelings by taking his toy do you think this fight would have started?"

"Of course not," Austin said.

"Why not?" I asked.

He said, "Because I wouldn't have had hurt feelings, and Mason would be feeling better."

I said, "I bet the reason Austin took the toy in the first place was that someone put dirt on his dish towel, so he got hurt feelings and was now mad at the world."

> Soon they realized that we are all inextricably connected and that we have a choice: we can express the truth of our relationships based on love or we can react violently to the hurt each other's feelings.

"In a big family like ours," I told them, "we have to learn how to express our own feelings and respect each other's feelings. I asked them, "Do you think people fight wars because they want to kill each other, or do you think someone gets hurt feelings and nobody listens? After people get hurt again and again, what do you think happens?"

They all said, "The people get mad and start a war."

I asked them, "What would you do to avoid a war like this?"

"We would ask the people who got their feelings hurt to tell us how they felt."

"Do you think that the people who were hurting those people realized that they were hurting them?"

The kids said, "Probably not, and if both sides could be truthful and tell each other how they really felt maybe they could be friends."

"It is hard to be truthful and tell your feelings, isn't it? But tell me how you feel now compared to when you were fighting."

They said they felt much better. I asked Mason, "Do you love your brother?" and he said, "Yes, I do."

Austin said, "I love you too, Mason. We're buddies."

I asked the kids to look at the dish towels we were holding and said, "If we keep putting dirt on these towels will we ever be able to love each other and enjoy being together? When you get hurt, your heart, which is the source of your feelings, shuts down. When you can't feel the love in your heart, you react with anger, and you hurt others along the way without realizing it, just like Mason did to me. Soon all of our relationships get dirty and then the relationships between you and your friends will become dirty. If your relationships become too dirty, you won't be able to get them clean again. The love and the communication that is in your hearts will be pushed further and further away until the only way you know how to be is just plain old mean and rotten."

Austin yelled, "Group hug!!!" and the crisis ended with big squeezes, and cleaner towels.

I am constantly using this technique, along with any other method I can think of, including bedtime stories and backyard soccer games, as opportunities to show them how their actions affect each other. Our soccer games get pretty intense, and every time we play, there is a lesson to be learned about how to communicate, and most importantly, how to be aware of how we make each other feel. Everyone wants to be loved—my goal is to convince them it is cool to show it.

Learning By Heart

Kids experience stress not only on the playground. Many children are finding that the classroom can be an even bigger "bear in the woods." Focusing in class and retaining information has become a real concern for our educational system.

Studies have reported that students retain:

- 10% of what they read
- 20% of what they hear
- 30% of what they see
- 50% of what they hear and see
- 70% of what they say
- 90% of what they say and DO

With the vast majority of teaching in American schools being simply verbal communication, kids don't really have a chance to retain what is expected of them. Traditional cultures always taught by example, by doing. Children might watch their dad work as a carpenter and want to imitate him. They might pick up some tools, as my children are always doing, and "play" with them. In this act of "doing" in the environment of play, kids learn. The fact of the matter is that not all kids learn in the same way. The Ayurvedic kid-types also describe learning styles.

Winter kid-types	learn best aurally (through sound)
Summer kid-types	learn best visually
Spring kid-types	learn best kinesthetically

Every child will learn aurally, visually and kinesthetically, but knowing your child's kid-type will help you identify the style of learning in which he or she will excel. As I describe these differences and some treatments for learning disorders, remember that children learn best in an atmosphere of play where they get to imitate you.

Winter Listening

Winter, or Vata, kid-types are sometimes restless and become easily over-stimulated, making it difficult for them to settle down, focus, and learn. Their minds naturally move quickly, and they learn best by listening because this is the fastest delivery system for transferring knowledge. When they are in balance they learn new information quickly and easily, but often have less skill retaining information. Their short-term memory banks see a lot of activity.

Summer Sight

Summer, or Pitta, kid-types are not likely to have learning difficulties. They are fiery, focused, driven, and competitive, and excel in our fast and furious society. They learn best visually and need to be able to read a book or see the blackboard to take advantage of their visual tendency. Because their nature is moderate in most things—somewhere between winter and spring—they have large accounts in both the short- and long-term memory banks.

Spring Movement

The spring, or Kapha, kid-types are generally easy-going, slow, and methodical, which carries over to their learning style. They often cannot cope with the rapid, auditory, lecture-based pace of the classroom. Once they do learn something, they retain the information or the knowledge for life, but they are slow to assimilate new information. This is particularly an issue when they in the slow spring cycle of their lives (up to age 12). They learn best when teaching is incorporated with movement, models, or objects they can manipulate, because the involvement of all their senses allows them to integrate the experience. They have what seems like limitless long-term memory banks but may have difficulty with short-term memory, making them seem forgetful.

Remember, rarely do you have a child who is predominantly one type. They usually are a combination of two kid-types, which both softens and rounds out the extreme tendencies of the single kid-types.

Learning Disorders in Kids

The two types of learning disorders that are described in Western science are: ADD (Attention Deficit disorder) and ADHD (Attention Deficit with Hyperactivity Disorder). If I were to generalize these disorders into the related kid-types, spring kid-types would be more likely to exhibit ADD and the winter and possibly summer kid-types would more likely to have ADHD. Until they reach their teens, all kids are in the heavy, slow spring lifecycle, so there is the tendency for any child with an improper diet, no exercise, and high levels of stress to develop attention deficit concerns.

> When we add up all the stress children are under today compared to the stress experienced by children of 30 years ago, it is no wonder that our children's nervous systems cannot settle down to study.

ADHD is usually related to constitutional tendencies that are exacerbated by environmental factors like social stress, diet, and nutrition. It is interesting that in Europe, where many of the lifestyle habits described in this book are still intact, the diagnosis of ADD is as rare today as it was in the United States 30 years ago. Currently in the U.S., 15% of school-age children are affected by attention deficit syndromes.

Let's look at the classic symptoms of both ADD and ADHD:

Attention Deficit Disorder

- Easily distracted
- Difficulty listening
- Difficulty focusing
- Disorganized
- Loses things easily
- Forgetful
- Can't seem to remain seated
- Talks excessively
- Poor study skills
- Works poorly alone

Attention Deficit Disorder with Hyperactivity

- High activity level
- Difficulty coping with change
- Aggressive behavior
- Socially immature
- Low self-esteem
- High frustration level
- Lack of control

Once you recognize these traits in your child, you can combine the information about the particular kid-type with the appropriate lifestyle recommendations and herbal treatments to optimally support your child's nervous system. But there are some specific key factors that have been recognized as being causative in ADD and ADHD.

Hereditary Causes

- Genetic—parents and grandparents
- Metal toxicity in mother—usually lead
- Birth trauma
- Prenatal alcohol and drug exposure

Allergy and Food Sensitivities

- Food additives
- Diet soft drinks with aspartame
- Food and cosmetic dyes
- Daily intake of: wheat, sugar, chocolate, oranges, yeast, malt, tap water, pesticides, and heavy metals
- Hormones in meats, milk, and eggs
- Heavy-metal poisoning when young—usually lead

Deficiencies

- Omega-3 fatty acids – marine lipids
- B-vitamins, vitamin C
- Magnesium, selenium, zinc, chromium, folic acid

Over-Stimulation

- Television
- Video games
- Internet
- Fast pace—shopping malls, traffic
- Irregular meals—fast food
- Action movies

When looking for help in treating ADD and ADHD, I recommend that you seek out a doctor who specializes in this area. These disorders are conditions that commonly result from the interaction of many complex factors. Look for someone who is willing to work with your child without using drugs as an initial treatment, but begins with diet, lifestyle, and herbal remedies. If these are not effective, then drugs may be an appropriate alternative. Generally speaking, there are some foods that contain specific micro-nutrients and minerals that are recommended for children with these types of issues.

These foods are:

- Whole grains
- Fresh vegetables
- Legumes
- Cold-water fish
- Organic meat
- Apricots
- Russet potatoes
- Broccoli

Essential oils that have balancing effects on the central nervous system are recommended by aromatherapists and Ayurvedic practitioners. They can be diffused in a child's bedroom at night while sleeping, or used in massage oil.

These essential oils are:

- Lemon balm (Melissa)
- Lavender
- Chamomile
- Rosemary

Naturopaths have had excellent results prescribing the amino acid glycine, which harmonizes and grounds the central nervous system. Glycine attaches to receptors in the central nervous system where it elicits a calming and balancing effect. The dosage used is 300–500 milligrams twice a day.

The Ayurvedic approach is to treat the whole individual by understanding the person's body type and treating the person accordingly. There is also a specific Ayurvedic herb that has been studied here in the West for its use with attention deficit disorders. It has proven to be an effective herbal remedy for many of the kids in my practice. It is always used as part of a comprehensive treatment package as the cause of the disorder or imbalance is almost always a complex combination of factors.

Bacopa Monniera

This herb's botanical name is *Bacopa monniera,* and although it is sometimes called *brahmi,* it is different from the North Indian herb also called *brahmi* or *gota kola.* Bacopa is one of the principal nerve tonics used in Ayurvedic medicine, and it is gaining notice in the West for the treatment of ADD and ADHD.

Bacopa has been traditionally used for improving memory and mental capacities in children. In recent years it has received attention for its reputation as a "brain tonic." Bacopa has been used for the treatment of epilepsy, nervous breakdowns, depression, and exhaustion. Its primary active constituents are called bacosides. These chemicals have been shown to alleviate fatigue, increase stamina, and enhance the metabolism of neurotransmitters, the chemical messengers between nerve cells, thereby increasing mental function. Bacosides may help to keep the toxic effects of stress to a minimum, and they have been shown to have antioxidant effects. Studies of subjects taking bacopa consistently demonstrate improved learning ability.

Bacosides have also been implicated in the improvement of short-term memory. *The Indian Journal of Psychiatry* reported in 2000 that bacopa significantly improved both short-term memory and learning in children between the ages of 8 and 10 years old taken at a dose of 50 milligrams twice a day. In 2002, *Neuropsychopharmacology* reported that taking bacopa produced significant effects on memory, especially the retention of information, in adults. Another study in *The Journal of Indian Drugs* that measured attention reported significant improvement in those people taking the herb. These results indicate that bacopa can be effective in attention deficit syndromes. No side effects or contraindications have been noted in the research with regard to children taking bacopa.

This herb, in conjunction with an overall approach specific to a child's kid-type to restore balance, can make huge strides in the treatment of ADD-related conditions.

The Heart of the Matter

All actions, thoughts, and desires originate in the heart, not the mind. The heart is the source of all our feelings and emotions. Because these feelings are so delicate, children quickly learn how to close off their hearts as a protective response. According to Vedic philosophy, the heart is the source of emotions and feelings as well as the spiritual center and Sacred Heart that gives access to one's own consciousness.

> The Upanishads, one of the most important Vedic texts, says that the heart is the faculty of thought.

According to the unified field theories of modern physics, all the matter and physical structures in the universe are described as being field-based. In other words, some of the tiniest particles of matter such as protons, neutrons, and electrons are just concentrated frequencies of the field and are not matter at all. The Vedic philosophy, from which Ayurveda comes, described this exact phenomenon over 5,000 years ago.

This consciousness that is the source of the human experience is said to be most concentrated in the heart. The heart, according to Ayurveda, is the source of *ojas,* the physical expression of consciousness. *Ojas* is a subtle substance in the body that controls immunity, reproduction, and spiritual and mental health.

> What the Vedic texts describe that modern physics has yet to discover is that this field is in fact our own consciousness.

Modern physiological research reveals a close connection among the heart and the brain and nervous system. According to research at the National Institutes of Health, 65% of the neurons found in the heart are identical to those found in the brain. The pericardium, the lining around the heart muscle, has also been shown to produce neurotransmitter chemicals which connect the heart to the nervous system. The heart is wired for more than just pumping blood—it is an organ with thinking and feeling potential as well.

Perhaps this explains why research suggests that only 5% of our lifelong learning is acquired from formal education, training, or schooling. That means 95% of a person's lifelong learning must come from somewhere else. According to the book, *Magical Parent, Magical child,* 95% of learning is state-specific. Researchers have discovered that if an experience is charged with an emotional quality or state of mind, the retention of the experience is greatly enhanced.

Batter Up!

Familiar smells can take us immediately to the realm of emotion and memory. One or two mornings each spring, I wake up to a particular smell in the air that brings me directly back to my Little League tryouts. When I was 10 years old, Little League tryouts was the most important day of my life. From the moment I opened my eyes on that morning, I felt palpable sensation of excitement, anxiety, and anticipation. Even now, years later, the crispness and smell of a baseball field's damp grass in spring can trigger those old emotions. Because the sense of smell (discussed in Chapter 10), directly accesses the structures of the limbic or emotional system of the brain through the olfactory nerve, certain smells can trigger very old and even forgotten memories.

Emotionally charged experiences can become lifelong memories that reside in our subconscious until we run across the same scent or emotional trigger, thereby bringing the memory of the experience back to the conscious part of the brain. It is true that we are wired to remember feelings of safety or danger as a part of the mechanisms for our own survival, and it is true that the most effective learning experience occurs in an environment of safety, calm, and comfort.

This kind of learning starts from the moment of conception, according to ancient traditions and Ayurvedic medicine. For thousands of years in Asia and India, safe, nurturing, and peaceful environments were created for expectant mothers in order to enhance this learning process. New studies show that if an expectant mother feels safe, the development of the baby's forebrain, which is the conscious, thinking area of the brain that controls creative capacities, will be enhanced. If the mother is stressed or threatened during pregnancy, the hindbrain, which is responsible for fight-or-flight survival functions, will be enhanced.

If the expectant mother is exposed to violence, stress, fear, jealousy, anger, and rage from watching television or movies, or even to the level of stress in our lives that has become an accepted part of our culture, the impact on the fetus and child is well documented.

Studies at Harvard University clearly show the importance of early bonding between mother and child as it relates to health and the ability for the child to interact socially. According to Alan Shore, Ph.D., the author of *Affective Regulation and the Origin of the Self*, it is in first 18 months of life that the self-image, intelligence, and socialization skills of the child are developed. The environment created by the parents during these first 18 months of life along with the previous 9 months of pregnancy may be the most important 27 months of that child's entire life.

> There is saying in Ayurveda: "what you see you become."

At the Institute of HeartMath, research in a new branch of cardiology called neurocardiology measured the electromagnetic field created by the heartbeat. Each phase of the heartbeat creates a unique and distinct field around the heart. The first phase creates a field close to the heart, followed by the next phase, which radiates a field approximately 3 feet from the heart. The third and final phase of the heartbeat radiates a field 12 to 15 feet from the body.

These fields can resonate with other people and are present in each and every relationship that we have. This may explain why you can be immediately attracted to a person or instantly know that a person is just not your type. This instantaneous knowledge may occur as a result of the harmony and resonance created by the electromagnetic field or the frequency coming from your own heart combined with the electromagnetic field from the heart of the other person.

These fields not only connect us with each other, they connect family members, especially a mother and her baby. Groundbreaking research done at Adelaide University in Australia discloses that cellular imprinting of the mother's heartbeat begins at conception and continues throughout the child's development. Current research emphasizes the importance of the resonance of the heartbeats between mother and child.

The bonding created during these first 18 months of the child's life between mother and child, as measured through their resonance field effects, supports a growing body of evidence that older cultural methods of child rearing are not only steeped in tradition but are also on the cutting edge of modern science. This research supports the importance of touch and closeness in the bond between mother and child.

It is theorized that mothers and their adopted children can entrain their heartbeat fields to create the necessary supportive environment for the child's optimal learning and development. Most importantly, it seems that the infant needs to have a constant and consistent, loving heart field in which to entrain and flourish. This is a new field of research, and only a small flake has been chipped from the iceberg of this knowledge.

Separating the child or infant from the mother or adopted mother for any length of time during these precious 18 months can create an unstable and incoherent field effect. The exact frequency of the field created by the resonance of the mother's and infant's heartbeats is precise and unique to those individuals, something akin to how animal mothers to recognize their offspring by their unique smell or voice. This field effect creates coherence in the brain of the infant, rich in harmony and love, with access to the higher states of learning that may offer us the keys to our human potential.

> The bond between these two electromagnetic heart fields sets up an environment of peace and calm, providing optimal learning as well as lifelong health for the child.

In traditional cultures where the mother, baby, and father sleep together in the same bed during the first years of the child's life, the incidence of crib death or sudden infant death syndrome (SIDS) is almost nonexistent. Where there are no cribs there is no crib death. Taking a child or infant away from the mother and putting him or her into a crib breaks the resonant field between them, setting up an emergency biochemistry of abandonment and fear for the infant. The non-intellectual, nonverbal bonding that takes place between mother and infant in the protective cocoon of their heart field is the best education a child will ever receive.

Have you ever noticed how people are attracted to infants and babies and how adults turn inside out when playing with a baby? An infant will interact with the mother and anyone else who comes into its focus with an experience of direct heart-to-heart communication. Perhaps that is why adults just can't seem to keep their eyes off a joyful baby. For the first two years of life, mother and infant communicate from moment to moment without a spoken word. Their communication is directly from the heart. This is also the time when Delta waves predominate in children's brains. Their minds are in a complete state of relaxation, allowing their joyful experience of the world to shine through in their communication with others.

The senses of speech, sight, and hearing that develop rapidly after the first 18 months of life change how growing infants interact with their world. As children age and the senses develop, they begin to filter this direct heartfelt communication, and ultimately the mind takes over.

Inevitably, as a child develops, exposure to mild stress and some emotional trauma are natural. The role of parents is to keep the road of emotional development free from any major traumatic events that could affect the child's long-term development.

> The extent to which children are protected from trauma and bond with their mothers on an energetic level is directly related to the mental and emotional health the children will enjoy as adults and the success they will experience in their spiritual development.

As the senses develop, feeling-based communication that results from the heart field resonance between the mother and child is replaced by the mind, via the development of the senses. A new personality created by the ego is set up to support the functioning of the mind and to maintain the protection of the vulnerable heart. No child wants to get hurt feelings, so the senses gracefully develop and the mind creates a personality designed to facilitate intellectual functioning and protect the child's feelings from being hurt. Soon the heart, which was the child's only means of communication, is replaced by communication through the senses, mind, and intellect. The heart, the feelings, and the original joy of an infant wait patiently to be reopened as part of the child's spiritual development later in life.

Albert Einstein having said that he used less than 10% of his brain potential might make us wonder how someone who made such great intellectual and personal achievements in his lifetime believed that he used such a small proportion of his mental and human potential. This means that the rest of us are no doubt leaving *more* than 90% of our conscious human potential untapped. In Ayurvedic medicine, this untapped potential is housed in the non-thinking, less-conscious areas of our brain. The part of the brain that is directly connected to our emotions and to our heart is what makes up the vast majority of our unrealized human potential.

If an individual is in a stressful environment, the thinking, intellectual, and survival-based part of the brain remains active. As the body becomes more peaceful and relaxed, the brain waves slow and become more coherent, just as we saw in the last chapter when the students were nasal breathing during exercise.

The more coherent brain-wave patterns, such as those seen in an Alpha state, are the patterns less of cognitive thinking and more of feeling-based mental activity. It is while experiencing these non-thinking states that humans report peak experiences in life.

When Roger Bannister broke the barrier of the four-minute mile in 1959, it was a feat that, at the time, was considered to be physically impossible. After he passed through the seemingly unbreakable barrier he said, "We seemed to be going so slowly....I was relaxing so much that my mind seemed detached from my body. There was no strain. There was no pain. Only a great unity of movement and aim. The world seemed to stand still or even not exist."

Athletes who experience this state of being call it "the zone." It is never experienced as a result of struggle and pain. It is always felt during a peak experience when a runner's best race is their easiest race, when world records are set with comfort and euphoria. In my book, *Body, Mind, and Sport,* I described a study in which we measured brain-wave function during runners' high experiences. The result revealed, as the athletes so clearly told us, that the zone is a state of effortless flow that requires no pain and no strain.

The "no pain-no gain" credo, which is still alive and well, will change only if we teach our children that life does not have to be a struggle. This will happen slowly, over time, and by our example. The road to perfect health merges the emotional, physical, mental, and even spiritual aspects of our potential into one large super-highway. Good physical health, which starts during childhood, is a prerequisite for a mentally and emotionally stable adult.

Less Is More

We have all had those feeling that when we struggle and try to accomplish something through force, we just can't seem to make it happen, but then when we relax the effort, it seems easy. It is like the children's woven fingercuff toy. You start out by placing one finger in each end of the woven tube, and then the trick is that you have to remove your fingers again. But if you try to remove them forcibly, no matter how hard you tug, they will not budge. It is only when you relax the effort that your fingers slide out again. In yoga, it is said that a true pose, or *asana,* is achieved only with steadiness and ease, not with effort. Similarly, the achievement of meditative states is reached without effort. These are states of mind when the thoughts do not dominate, but there exists quiet awareness.

> The zone described by athletes is a state of mind that can be reached only through relaxing the effort. Almost all scientists agree that the harder you try to get into the zone, the less likely it is that you will.

The Zone Is Like the Quiet in the Eye of the Storm

Billie Jean King, who wrote the foreword to *Body, Mind, and Sport,* said it best about her peak experiences while playing tennis:

> "I would transport myself beyond the turmoil of the court to a place of total peace and calm."

The evidence is clearly mounting in support of the theories that suggest that human potential—the 90% of our physical, emotional, mental, and spiritual capacity that we do not currently access—will come from a feeling-based, non-thinking experience and state-of-being, rather than the intellectual efforts and struggles of the conscious mind.

> According to the philosophy of yoga, the quality of the breath influences how the mind will react in any situation: either in a thinking-based state of emergency or in a relaxed feeling-based state of calm.

In the previous chapter, I discussed the effects that nasal breathing while exercising and sleeping has on facilitating the neurological calm and slower brain-wave activity that support the chemistry of play and allow us to access our true potential. Mouth breathing, on the other hand, supports an emergency-based, constricting neuro-chemistry that robs vital energy from the brain—not enough breath can enter the body through the tightly held-in lungs. As long as oxygen levels remain relatively low, the brain will trigger an increased amount of fight or flight survival-oriented activity.

When you or your children breathe through the nose, the efficiency of oxygen intake and carbon dioxide release is improved. The more oxygen the brain receives, the more the protective survival-based emergency response is replaced with a feeling-based experience from

> If we can train our children to handle most of life's stressful situations with equanimity, ease, and steadiness, it will create an environment in their biochemistry of safety and peace, allowing them to feel inner love and experience optimal learning.

the heart. In Chapter 10, this experience was measured by the change in brain-wave production with nasal breathing from incoherent Beta waves to coherent Alpha waves during exercise. With this change, the incessant activity and constant thoughts of the mind are quieted.

John and Beatrice Lacey, after 30 years of research for the National Institutes of Health, found a direct neural connection between the heart and the brain. Our feeling and thoughts are anatomically hard-wired together but we do not always experience a clear connection between them. When breathing is shallow and life is stressful, oxygen levels in the brain are low or merely adequate and the connection between the brain and heart is compromised. With full and deep nasal breathing and a nurturing environment, the child's brain can be fully integrated as a whole, utilizing all of its capacity; and the connection between brain and heart can be reforged and solidified, giving access to fully integrated physical and mental health. Much of this pavement is laid during the first 18 months of life and the previous 9 months of embryonic development in the womb.

> The lake becomes still and the mind becomes clear with direct access to the feelings and emotions of the heart...the vault to our human potential has been unlocked.

An Ayurvedic Perspective

Ayurveda describes a subtle approach to our physiology which emphasizes the need to nurture the developing child and protect the mother during pregnancy. According to Ayurveda, conception initiates the development of the new individual's subtle bodies, called Koshas (which means sheaths). These subtle bodies, described in detail some 5,000 years ago, may be related to the heart fields of modern science. The subtle field that is located within and connected to the body surrounds it, measuring up to 15 feet in diameter, just like the electromagnetic heart fields measured with each heartbeat. Ayurvedic and yogic philosophies delineate this field into five subtle bodies or five layers. The purpose of these five Koshas is to support the development of the person beginning at conception and continuing throughout life, ultimately supporting the individual's spiritual process.

These five sheaths manifest from the unified field previously mentioned. This field, according to Ayurveda, is our own consciousness. It is the creative spiritual life force, *shakti,* or love, that fuels life itself. After conception, the mother and child together create an electromagnetic or heart field, which supports the progressive development of the subtle bodies into matter and a physical body. These sheaths develop around the source, pure consciousness, like the layers of an onion.

The following is a description of the five sheaths and their functions in development and throughout our lives:

- At the center of this field is pure consciousness, the creative source from which everything arises, known as *Atman.*
- The center field of pure consciousness, *kundalini shakti,* connected to the source is protected by the first subtle body known as *Anandamaya Kosha,* or the sheath of bliss. It is sometimes called the causal body because it causes the creation of the next four sheaths.
- The second sheath is that of intellect and discernment, called the *Vijnanamaya Kosha.* The functions of this sheath include: pure intellect and understanding without emotion, the intrinsic knowledge of good and bad, and direct access to source.
- The third sheath, also called the great barrier sheath, is the mental sheath, or *Manomaya Kosha.* This sheath of the mind contains desire, memories, ego, and emotion. It is here that we can become disconnected from our access to the source.
- The fourth sheath is the energy sheath, or *Pranamaya Kosha.* This sheath regulates the flow of subtle energy in the body. It uses prana (subtle energy), the nadis (subtle nerve flow), and chakras (subtle energy centers) to transform thought into action, allowing the mind to affect and direct the body.

- The fifth sheath is the sheath of the gross or material body, the *Annamaya Kosha*. This sheath is the physical manifestation of the previous four subtle bodies and gives us our physical form.

These sheaths begin with the source of consciousness and culminate with the manifestation of the physical body. They are created sequentially from the inside out, from the subtle to the material. Since the heart field is the center of our consciousness, it is critical for this process. The coherence and sanctity of children's heart fields progress them through the developmental stages that will directly affect their health, well-being, and spiritual processes. The goal of the sciences of Ayurveda and yoga is to support and balance the subtle bodies so that when a child or an adult begins a spiritual life it will be a successful one. Ayurveda and yoga were created for this purpose—not only for physical health and longevity, but also for the successful pursuit of a spiritual life and the achievement of our full potential as human beings.

Here in the West, we often use yoga merely as a physical and mental health tool and are often unaware that each posture carries a specific vibrational frequency designed to direct or redirect the pure consciousness fully and effectively through these five sheaths. The practices of Ayurveda and the achievement of perfect physical health prepare the body to be able to support this spiritual process. Success is achieved when the mind gives up its control to the heart—and the heart regains its natural role as the faculty of all thoughts, actions, and desires.

> When we fully unite body, mind, spirit and breath, we play from the heart, on the playground of love, naturally developing our full human potential.

I am a firm believer that there is nothing that our human body cannot do—within reason, of course. I also believe that the stress we endure in our daily lives is the biggest inhibitor of our enjoyment of our lives and our ability to tap into the full human potential that awaits us. Many traditional health care systems have mapped out the road to this dormant potential inside of us. In this book I share the health secrets that have changed the way we raise our children. I also introduce you to a system of medicine designed to prepare you and your children for the human potential that waits patiently in the depths of all of our hearts and minds.

> If we are to have real peace, we must begin with the children.
> —Gandhi

Index

347

About the Author

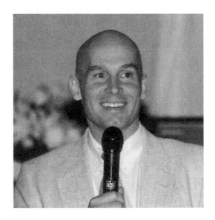

After studying Ayurveda in the West, Dr. Douillard went to India in 1986 for a three-week vacation. During his visit, he was invited to stay on permanently to learn Ayurveda first-hand from a master teacher.

Without hesitation, he closed his Colorado practice via phone and remained in India for more than a year, undertaking the first phase of his Ayurvedic education abroad.

Near the end of this period in India, he met Dr. Deepak Chopra, who invited him to become the Associate Director of his Ayurvedic Center in Massachusetts.

In that capacity, Dr. Douillard became the Co-Director of the Physicians Training Program, where he certified Western medical doctors in Ayurvedic medicine for eight years.

Dr. Douillard continued extensive training in India and received his Ph.D. in Ayurvedic medicine from the Open International University in Sri Lanka.

A former professional athlete, Dr. Douillard published his first book, *Body, Mind, and Sport* (which has sold over 60,000 copies and is printed in six languages) in 1992.

Seven years later, he was hired by the New Jersey Nets NBA team as their Director of Player Development. In 2000, he published his second book, *The 3-Season Diet*. His fourth book, *The LifeSpa Ayurvedic Massage Manual,* is due to be released in January 2004.

Dr. Douillard has produced two audio-cassette series, *Invincible Athletics* and *Ayurvedic Pulse Reading*. He has developed a preservative-free Ayurvedic skin-care line and has recently launched an Ayurvedic herbal line for health professionals.

He has been teaching Ayurveda internationally for fifteen years and specializes in pulse reading, Ayurvedic fitness, and Panchakarma.

Currently, he practices Ayurvedic and chiropractic medicine at his LifeSpa in Boulder, Colorado, where he lives with his wife and six children.

For more information about Dr. Douillard's books, tapes, and lectures, or training schedules, services, and programs, please contact:

LifeSpa
PO Box 701
Niwot, CO 80544
Office: 303.516.4848
Fax: 303.530.4409
E-mail: *John@LifeSpa.com*
Website: *www.LifeSpa.com*

John Douillard's
LifeSpa Programs and Services

Educational Materials
Books:

The 3-Season Diet: Eat the way nature intended

Body, Mind, and Sport: The mind-body guide to lifelong health, fitness, and your personal best

The LifeSpa Ayurvedic Massage Training Manual: In press; expected publication: Spring 2004

Other:

Invincible Athletics: This audio series is similar to *Body, Mind, and Sport* with more emphasis on Ayurveda

Pulse Reading Course: This course will take you step by step into an understanding of Ayurveda and pulse diagnosis.

Products
Complete herbal line

Preservative-free skin care products

Books and tapes written by Dr. Douillard

Services
Panchakarma

Dayspa treatments

Chiropractic

Ayurvedic consultations

Telephone consultations

Education
Ayurvedic massage training

Body, Mind, and Sport Personal Trainer certification

The 3-Season Diet weight loss programs

LifeSpa's Ayurvedic online training programs for health care professionals—free with wholesale accounts.

www.LifeSpa.com

Convenient online ordering

Medicine Chest: Determine which herbs are best for your condition and take an active role in your own healing. Descriptions, links to articles, recommended dosages, precautions, and purchasing are included.

Library: Find articles written by Dr. John Douillard on subjects such as diet, health conditions, and many others.

Many other resources to support optimal health and well-being